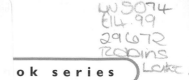
Working with Family Carers

A guide to good practice

Jacqui Wood and Phill Watson

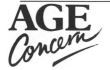

BOOKS

© 2000 Jacqui Wood and Phill Watson

Published by Age Concern England
1268 London Road
London SW16 4ER

First published 2000

Editor Gillian Clarke
Design and typesetting GreenGate Publishing Services
Production Vinnette Marshall
Printed in Great Britain by Bell & Bain Ltd, Glasgow

A catalogue record for this book is available from the British Library.

ISBN 0-86242-230-2

Bulk orders
Age Concern England is pleased to offer customised editions of all its titles to UK companies, institutions or other organisations wishing to make a bulk purchase. For further information, please contact the Publishing Department at the address on this page. Tel: 020 8765 7200. Fax: 020 8765 7211. E-mail: addisom@ace.org.uk.

CONTENTS

Appendix 2

ABOUT THE AUTHORS

Jacqueline Wood's first experience of caring came when her grandmother developed Alzheimer's disease. The illness itself was distressing enough for the whole family, but the situation was made worse initially by the lack of information and support. Fortunately, her family was able to share the work of caring but this is not often the case for carers. The responsibility usually falls to one person.

When Jacqui began her career in the field of care, she was sometimes in conflict with carers, because she worked in the interest of people with learning disabilities, which was not always compatible with their parents' wishes. However, she quickly came to realise – through the early days of consultation and the development of community care – that the concept of enabling people to continue to live in their own home means additional responsibilities for many of their family members. The contribution made by carers is vital to the success of community care.

Phill Watson completed a BA Honours degree in Sociology and Social Policy at the University of Sheffield, and then trained as a registered general nurse at the Sheffield School of Nursing. After working at King's College Hospital, London, he began working in the voluntary sector, as the Disabled Living Services Manager with the Association for Spina Bifida and Hydrocephalus.

From 1992 to January 1998, Phill worked for Carers National Association, as Assistant Director, Development. At Carers National Association he was closely involved with the increasing recognition of the role of carers and the need to ensure that people working with carers are properly informed and supported.

Currently Phill is Chief Officer with Age Concern Bexley.

ACKNOWLEDGEMENTS

The authors thank the many carers, friends and colleagues for their invaluable help and advice in producing this book. In particular:

Kent's carers' workers, who have developed so many excellent ways to support carers and whose knowledge was drawn upon.

West Kent Social Services care managers for providing such explicit insights into assessments for service users and carers.

Hampshire Social Services, and especially Geoff Woolen for his wisdom and common-sense approach.

Helen Ferguson, Co-ordinator for Carers National Association, Northern Ireland.

Alan McGuinley, Co-ordinator for Carers National Association, Scotland.

National Information Forum.

Cicely Northcote Trust.

Elgar Housing Association, Worcestershire.

Social Services Inspectorate.

The Information and Advice team at Carers National Association head office in London.

In addition we thank all the national organisations that support carers, and whose materials and information have ensured that the book will be a valuable and authentic resource for care professionals. We are grateful to Carers National Association for permission to reproduce the self-assessment form on pages 29 and 30.

A 'thank you' also to the people at Age Concern who offered their guidance throughout the writing of this book.

INTRODUCTION

This handbook has been written with two people in mind: the carer and the face-to-face care worker. It is designed to address the concerns of both.

In recent years there has been a growing awareness of the important role played by carers and the fact that they are the mainstay of community care. At the same time, the face-to-face care worker finds that there are ever-increasing demands for services but limited resources with which to deliver them.

There has probably never been a more appropriate time for this handbook for professionals, whose greatest resource may well be carers themselves. It is for this reason that professionals must see carers as partners rather than as potentially another user group.

Whether you are a qualified, experienced social worker, a medical practitioner or a student, this book will help you to understand the challenges that carers face and your part in supporting them through those challenges. Although it cannot provide solutions to every problem you are likely to encounter, it gives some practical tips and experiences that may be helpful when adapted to your own situation.

We look only briefly at the management of services with their policies and strategies, because this is very much a book for people working at the practical end. The 'hands-on' workers have the opportunity of experiencing the reality of caring every day through the service user or patient and the carer. They hear of the anger and frustrations of carers struggling to make ends meet, find their way through the maze of information that might or might not be helpful to them, maintain their own health and look after a close relative or friend.

It is you, the face-to-face worker, who sees the pain and anguish a carer can go through as they watch someone they love become more ill or disabled. It is you who can make a difference to these situations and help carers bring some positive aspects into their own lives and the lives of the people they care for.

This book encourages you to know about services and sources of support, and suggests how you might do this. It will not be your job to do everything for everyone. However, if your network is well developed, you will be able to deal with many of the requests you get from carers or refer them to someone who can. The book also looks at what to do when it is not possible to act on a carer's request arising from an assessment.

We look at the practical issues of caring, including financial difficulties, conflict, and emotional and physical stress. The Carers (Recognition and Services) Act 1995 is also described in some detail, explaining what it means for carers and how you can ensure that their rights are maintained.

We hope you will use this handbook as a working guide, drawing on the ideas and suggestions and developing your ability to 'think carer' in a creative way. Take up the invitation to see your relationship with carers grow into mutual respect and support as partners in care.

1 You and carers – a partnership

Carers – who are they?

'A carer is someone looking after a friend, relative or neighbour who cannot manage without help because of sickness, age or disability.'
Carers National Association

The 1990 General Household Survey revealed that one person in seven was a carer (46 per cent were aged 45–59 and 28 per cent were aged 60 or over). This means that there are more than 6.8 million carers in the UK. Many more are former carers, or will become carers in the very near future. The figures do not include young carers under the age of 18, of whom there are between 15,000 and 40,000 (research published by the Health Services Management Unit at Manchester University in 1995 estimated the figure to be 40,000).

Carers are ordinary people, often carrying extraordinary responsibilities. They are of every age, culture, class and religion. They are wives, husbands, partners, parents, children, other relatives and friends. Most carers are women, but a large minority (43 per cent) are men.

The 1990 General Household Survey also found that 23 per cent of carers were spending more than 20 hours a week caring and that 11 per cent were spending more than 50 hours a week. Carers National Association wanted to find out in much more detail what it is like to be a carer and what effect caring has on the lives of carers, so in 1992 it commissioned a survey of its members. The results were published under the title *Speak Up, Speak Out*. They make disturbing reading:

- 47 per cent of Carers National Association members have had financial difficulties since becoming a carer;
- 65 per cent say that their own health has suffered;
- 20 per cent have never had a break;
- 33 per cent get no help or support with their caring responsibilities.

Some of the comments that carers made in *Speak Up, Speak Out* sum up these problems:

'I'm depressed and hopeless, and the lack of sleep is terrible.'

'I want financial improvements for us so that we are not made to feel like beggars.'

'I'd like a night's sleep – absolutely unbroken – every two weeks or so.'

For some, caring is a job they do 24 hours a day, seven days a week.

According to the Institute of Actuaries, carers provide support worth £34 billion each year, which would otherwise have to be found by the state. Many do not recognise themselves as carers, partly because about three-quarters of the 6.8 million provide care for fewer than 20 hours a week. They are often providing help and support of a practical nature such as shopping, housework and cooking for the dependent person, and so do not see it as 'care' even though it can be tiring and time consuming. It could be argued that many women would be doing these tasks in any case, but we must remember that a significant number of carers are men who might not normally be so involved or that there are women caring at a distance and therefore have their own housework to do in addition.

Carers may be involved in a wide range of caring responsibilities. These include:

- *Domestic chores*, such as cleaning, cooking, shopping.
- *Personal care*, such as washing, dressing, toileting the person.
- *Medical care*, such as giving medicines or injections, changing colostomy bags.
- *Emotional support* to the person being cared for.

There has been much debate about the figures estimated for caring. After all, can a few hours of caring each week really be costed? As

Baroness Pitkeathley, former Chief Executive of the Carers National Association, once said 'Caring for a few hours a week may not seem very significant to some, but it may be those few hours that is helping someone stay in their own home rather than entering residential accommodation.'

In the report *Community Care: Agenda for action* (1988), the late Sir Roy Griffiths wrote :

'A failure to give proper levels of support to informal carers not only reduces their own quality of life and that of the relative and friend they care for, but it is also potentially inefficient as it can lead to less appropriate care being offered. Positive action is therefore needed to encourage the delivery of more flexible support which takes account of how best to support and maintain the role of the informal carer.'

Raised awareness

Since that report, considerable progress has been made for carers. There is greater awareness of the contribution they make. Much media attention is given to the subject and it is without doubt firmly established on the social and political agenda. The discussions and statements made in preparation for the National Health Service and Community Care Act 1990 raised the expectations of carers. In 1990 Virginia Bottomley, then Health Minister, said:

'Although not enshrined in legislation, the role of carers most clearly will be given the priority they deserve in all our guidance about assessment, about community care plans and about all other aspects of these proposals.'

The National Health Service and Community Care Act 1990 emphasises consultation and negotiation, encourages collaboration between agencies and requires assessment of a person's needs and consultation with the carer. The Carers (Recognition and Services) Act 1995 requires local authorities to carry out a separate assessment of the carer. They must take the results of the assessment into account when deciding on the level of service to be provided to the person being cared for.

However, in *Better Tomorrows?*, commissioned in 1995 by Carers National Association, Norman Warner revealed that four out of five carers think that community care changes have made no difference to them, or even that services have deteriorated. As many as one in four carers may be experiencing hardship as a result of increased charges for services, and over 60 per cent of carers did not know that they can ask for a separate assessment of their own needs.

The experiences of the people below are not unusual.

CASE STUDY

Ann and **Bill** are a pensioner couple who live in Liverpool. Ann has Parkinson's disease, and recently was admitted to hospital. When she was discharged she was told that, although her care needs had increased substantially, the social services department could pay only £100 a week towards her home care. At Bill's request, the £100 budget is used to provide overnight care two nights a week (but he has to pay an extra £12 a week, as the cost is actually £112). Bill can't manage without more help but he has been told that either Ann will have to go into a nursing home or he will have to cope as best he can.

CASE STUDY

Carol and **Don** live in Lancashire. Carol looks after Don, who, like Ann, has Parkinson's disease. To see whether Don could manage without medication, his doctor stopped it; three days later Don was admitted to hospital as an emergency case. He was in shock and unable to pass water. After seven weeks in hospital, Don was sent home suddenly one morning, although Carol could see no improvement. She now struggles to look after him. One day he fell out of the chair and she had to get two passing strangers to lift him back. No one called that day. That night the twilight nurse called at 11pm and arranged for him to be readmitted to hospital as an emergency.

CASE STUDY

Emma, who lives in the West Midlands, told us about her parents, **Frank** and **Gloria**. Frank, 82, looks after Gloria, 86, who has Alzheimer's disease. Frank had a heart attack and was admitted to hospital. Gloria was also admitted because no alternative care was available. They were discharged with no extra support – Emma was not consulted or even notified. The social services department told Emma that her parents were not coping after discharge and that either she would have to look after them or they would have to go into a home. They do not want to go into a home but Emma has mental health problems herself and feels unable to take full responsibility for her parents' care.

It is no wonder that carers in *Speak Up, Speak Out* said about caring:

'It's bloody awful and gets worse by the week.'

'It's not something I would have taken on full time if I had known then what I know now. Not a life I would wish on my worst enemy.'

'It's the worst wearing job in the world – with no light at the end of the tunnel. My husband is very deaf, can't see well – so there's not much conversation – one does feel lonely.'

Why do carers care?

Caring can start suddenly: for example, when a previously healthy and able person has a stroke or heart attack or is injured in a fall or accident. For many people, though, the role of caring develops gradually, when someone becomes increasingly ill, frail or disabled. Because it can be so gradual, carers do not at first recognise that they are taking on the caring role. Neither do they recognise at what stage help may be needed, whether for themselves or the person they are caring for. As the situation becomes worse, carers realise that they need information about what help may be available, but by this stage they are often too exhausted to deal with the inevitable bureaucracy involved with both statutory and voluntary agencies.

CASE STUDY

Janet is married with two teenage sons. She used to work full-time as a secretary in an estate agent's office. Until three years ago, her mother, at 62, was active and independent even though she had occasional pain because of the onset of arthritis. When her mother was going through a bad patch, Janet would help her out by going over to her house at the week-ends and doing the housework her mother found more difficult, such as cleaning windows, moving furniture for a good monthly cleaning and changing the bed linen.

As time went by, Janet noticed that her mother was beginning to lose weight and didn't seem to get out and about as much as she used to. Janet discovered that the arthritis was beginning to get worse, so she persuaded her mother to see the GP. Newly prescribed drugs helped for a while, but the bouts of pain were starting to cause some depression.

To make sure her mother was eating properly, Janet drove to her house most evenings to cook her a meal. At the week-ends she would bring her mother back to her own home for Saturday and Sunday lunch. This created additional tension in her own family, as there never seemed to be any time to spend with her husband at week-ends, and they were both at work through the week.

Within a year, Janet was also having to drive to her mother's every morning before going to work, to help her get up and dressed. She had arranged for some help during the day, but her mother liked to get up at 7am and she could not find anyone willing to be available early enough. Janet was beginning to feel permanently tired.

Eventually, Janet switched to part-time work even though it caused her family some problems financially. She felt it was the only way she could continue to help her mother and to stay healthy herself. Because of the depression, her mother went out less and less, and never seemed to be satisfied with the help she was given.

Janet became more and more frustrated with her situation but had no idea what to do about changing it. She'd not heard of the term 'carer' and didn't realise this is what she had become.

Carers sometimes get drawn into the caring role without meaning to. Perhaps they are the relative who lives nearest to the person needing care. Caring can begin out of feelings of guilt – for example, 'I couldn't put Mother into a home and there's no one else to look after her'. The experience of caring can often be governed by some or all of the following.

The quality of the relationship before the care started Caring for a person the carer did not much like can be extremely stressful for both carer and cared-for. However, previous affection can see both parties through the difficult times and help to make it a more rewarding experience.

The support networks available to the carer Whether carers are drawn into the situation gradually or suddenly, they need emotional, social and financial support to some degree. Lack of such support creates worry and tension, and a very negative experience of caring, as well as possibly leading to illness in the carers themselves.

The opportunity for a break Caring (particularly for long hours, day in and day out) will take its toll on carers if they do not receive regular respite. Moreover, a break from each other can be just as refreshing for the person being cared for.

Information about the condition of the person being cared for This is particularly relevant to carers of people with a mental health problem. For example, a doctor may feel that it is inappropriate to disclose medical information about a patient, but the carer needs to know certain facts to help in their caring.

KEY POINTS

- The caring role can develop gradually rather than the carer making a conscious decision to care.
- There are many reasons why people take up the caring role, and you should never make the assumption that it is solely through choice.
- Carers will feel more able to continue if they have support networks available to them.
- Regular respite can be a welcome break for both the carer and the person being looked after.

The carer and the professional

The term 'professional' is used frequently in this book to describe those who are responsible for providing help and support to people needing health, social or community services. It refers to those who are paid to do a job. It should be remembered that carers are unpaid professionals, having developed their abilities, knowledge and skills over many years of trial and error, often without support.

A partnership *with* carers can be nurtured only through listening and learning *from* carers. Yet while developing ways to work in partnership, the professional must bear in mind that carers may also need services.

'I look after Jayne, but who looks after me?' Widowed mother of a disabled young woman

Identifying a carer

Many carers do not realise what a vital role they play. Often, they are so used to being ignored that they shy away from expressing their feelings. This is particularly true when visiting the doctor with, or on behalf of, the person being cared for, but it is also true of many other encounters with professionals.

The following examples are ways in which carers may first be identified. It is our responsibility as health or social services professionals to ask ourselves certain questions.

- Someone is talking or writing to you about a relative, friend or neighbour needing help. [*Why are they involved? What do they do?*]
- A person seeking help may have someone with them or will happen to mention them in some way. [*Why are they there? What do they do for that person?*]
- Someone has applied for help at home for the first time and has been offered a service. [*How did they cope before? Do they need help at other times? Is anyone else providing services that cannot be given by social services?*]
- An older patient has severe mobility problems, and is becoming forgetful, but still manages to visit the doctor's surgery. [*How is that person managing at home? Who helps with the heavy household tasks? Who is reminding them to take their medicine?*]
- A school child is not succeeding as expected and is constantly tired. [*Why is this happening?*]

Until the questions are asked, it is unlikely that any answers will be found. Recognising a carer is the crucial first step. Until this is done, nothing else can follow. There is also a danger that, by providing help to the person needing care but not taking into account the needs of the carer, the carer's task will be made more difficult and frustrating.

KEY POINTS

- Many people do not recognise themselves as carers.
- It is up to the professionals to 'think carer' and ask relevant questions.
- Providing help to a service user or patient without taking account of the carer's needs can make their task more difficult.

Young carers

'Young carers' are children and young people under the age of 18 years whose lives are in some way restricted because they have to take responsibility for the care of a person who is ill, has a disability, is experiencing mental distress or is affected by substance misuse.

Most young carers are caring for a parent, commonly in a single-parent family, but some may be responsible for a grandparent, sibling or other family member. Some may be the primary carer – the only person providing care – but others may be secondary carers, sharing responsibilities with other family members.

HOW MANY YOUNG CARERS ARE THERE?

Research published by the Health Services Management Unit at Manchester University in 1995 indicates that there may be up to 40,000 young carers nationally. Accurate figures are difficult to obtain. In our experience, young carers and their parents are often silent about the extent of caring because they are afraid of being separated or from guilt, pride or a desire to 'keep it in the family'. Identifying young carers from minority ethnic groups can be even more difficult, because of differing cultural and religious needs.

WHAT ARE THE EFFECTS ON YOUNG CARERS?

Their caring responsibilities may result in lateness and absenteeism from school. They are often tired and find it difficult to concentrate on schoolwork. As a result, they may not achieve their full potential or be able to go on to further education because of their caring responsibilities. There is a strong likelihood that, because the parent is ill and cannot work, the family will be on a low income or receiving state benefits. This compounds the loss of educational and career opportunities that many young carers face. They can also suffer from the stigma that may be perceived by their peers because of a home life that is different from other people's. This difficulty in relationships with their peers may be even greater if a young person is caring for someone with a mental health problem, is addicted to drugs or alcohol or has HIV or an AIDS-related illness.

All these factors result in the loss of childhood, affecting a child physically, emotionally, educationally and socially, and causing scars that may be carried into adulthood.

> 'Everyone mentions different things people are entitled to and the rights they should get. The greatest right is the right to be a child, and that's what gets taken away.' Young carer, Sefton

WHAT YOU CAN DO

- Increase your awareness of the needs of young people with caring responsibilities.
- Raise awareness of this issue among colleagues.
- Include provision for young carers when planning future services.
- Listen, believe and respond to young carers with whom you come into contact.
- Provide young carers with understandable, relevant information that may help them.
- Be aware of who is providing care when assessing or discussing the needs of the sick or disabled person.
- Explore with young carers and their families the choices available and the practical assistance that may be of use to them.
- Initiate and encourage developments that aim to improve the lives of young carers.
- Promote the rights of young carers as both children and carers.
- Revise training programmes to ensure a sensitive and consistent response from staff.

KEY POINTS

- A fear of separation and a desire to 'keep it in the family' can lead to young carers remaining 'hidden'.
- Although most young carers are caring for a parent, some care for a grandparent or other family member.
- A young carer's social, physical, educational and emotional development can be affected because of their caring role.
- Young carers need information, practical support and someone to talk to.

The difficulties faced by carers

Many carers find that their health suffers because of exhaustion and stress. Physical problems can arise, such as back pain from having to support or lift the person being cared for, often with no training on how to do this safely. Continuous nights of broken sleep are common, particularly for carers of people with dementia. This can lead to increased stress, tiredness and, as a result, low resistance to illness.

'If I could just get one night of unbroken sleep every couple of weeks, I think I would cope much better.' Carer of someone with dementia

Caring causes financial hardship too, not only because of the costs of providing care such as extra laundry, higher heating bills, special diets, etc, but also because the carers often have to give up a job to provide the care that is needed. Some might argue that Attendance Allowance is provided to cover such costs. In reality, though, this often falls short of the cost of caring, and does not take account of the loss of earned income. As well as affecting income, this may have a serious effect on the carer's future security and pension. In *The True Cost of Caring*, a survey in 1996 by the Caring Costs Alliance, it was revealed that 56 per cent of carers faced future financial problems because they had lost the opportunity to build up savings or pension contributions.

Isolation and loneliness are also a problem for many carers, who can spend several days or weeks with the person they care for as their only company. This can be especially frustrating and isolating if the person being cared for has communication difficulties or dementia.

All of this presents a very negative view of caring, but it is a reality. However, with the right help and support, it can be a more rewarding and positive experience both for the carer and for the person receiving care.

Conflicts with the person needing support

It is important to understand that caring takes place in the context of a relationship, not all of which are based on openness, honesty, mutual respect and understanding. Crucially, in caring relationships there are differences from most other relationships. There is often little room for negotiation, possibly because the person being cared for may not be easy to negotiate with. Indeed, some people may be unreasonable in their expectations of the carer or in their willingness to accept support offered by outside agencies. In such instances it is important to recognise such conflicts and to help negotiate a better outcome and to support the carer in considering their needs as well as those of the person being cared for.

The conflicts for the person being cared for can be great. For some there is a desire for independence and for 'not being a burden', yet reconciling this with the right to have care delivered in a way that is acceptable while maintaining as normal a life as possible. It must be recognised that there may be a tendency for some carers to encourage dependence, because this can provide them with a sense of purpose and meaning. In such circumstances it may be that the relationship actively discourages people from developing independent life skills or impinges on the ability of someone to control their own life. This can lead to uncomfortable conflicts of loyalty for you. Should you support the carer or the person being cared for? If your reason for being there is to support the carer, that is where your loyalty should lie; if appropriate and possible, the person being cared for should be referred to an organisation that can act as an advocate for them.

Does the carer want to care?

Many carers would never consider any alternative to caring for the person they love, but it should not be assumed that all carers feel this way.

- Some will take up the caring role because of a sense of duty.
- Some minority ethnic cultures often expect the daughter or wife to undertake the caring role.
- Other carers are unaware that there might be another choice.
- Some carers will feel that they can manage only if they have some help in caring.

Whilst some carers have made their decision from the start, it may take a formal carer's assessment to help others to decide.

In some instances, carers may have wanted to take on this responsibility to start with, but find later that they can no longer cope and have changed their mind. Reasons for this include:

- The carer did not realise the level of care needed.
- The person being cared for has become more disabled or ill.
- The carer cannot afford to provide care and needs to earn an income.

- The carer was unaware of how much it would change their life; for example, losing touch with friends because of not being able to go out socially very often, or losing self-confidence because of stopping work.
- The carer's relationship with a partner is under stress because of caring.

Taking a decision not to care can be distressing and difficult for both the carer and the person being cared for. The carer needs support in understanding that it is their right to make that decision, just as it is the right of the person needing care to have the best choices available.

When a carer can no longer cope

Although many carers may reach a stage where they feel they cannot cope any longer, often the intervention of respite services and domiciliary help can change that situation. However, if the carer has come to the decision that they are no longer willing or able to look after someone else's care needs, they and the person they are caring for have to consider the alternatives available. The main option is likely to be residential care.

Local authority social services departments (social work departments in Scotland, or health and social services boards in Northern Ireland) vary in their policies on providing residential care, and you should know about these. Appendix 1 explains the local authority charging procedure for someone assessed as qualifying for residential care.

If a person does not qualify for financial help and is looking for private residential care, most social services departments can provide a list of registered homes even though they do not make recommendations. Similarly, the National Care Homes Association may be able to provide a list of local care homes that are affiliated to the Association; such homes must follow a standard of high quality services and adhere to the Association's code of conduct.

The carer and the person they are caring for will need support, and time to enable them to find the right home, in the right location and at the right price.

KEY POINTS

- More than half of all carers face financial problems.
- Caring can cause social isolation, as well as physical and emotional stress.
- Conflict between a carer and the person they are caring for should be seen as a normal part of caring. The professional worker can help people deal with those conflicts.
- Carers have the right to change their minds about decisions they made earlier.

Landmark legislation

The most important legislation relating to carers and community care is:

- National Assistance Act 1948 (section 21): a duty to accommodate ill, elderly and disabled people
- Health Services and Public Health Act 1968 (section 45): the power to provide community-based services for elderly people
- Chronically Sick and Disabled Persons Act 1970 (section 2): the duty to provide community-based services for disabled people
- National Health Service Act 1997 (section 8): a duty to provide community-based services for ill people

Under this legislation there was a duty to provide services after the social services department had decided that someone was in need of the them, but that department was not required to make that decision (what is now called an assessment). This meant that social services departments could bypass their duty to provide by simply not deciding (or assessing) whether someone needed services.

The Disabled Persons (Services, Consultation and Representation) Act 1986 (the Disabled Persons Act) was designed to overcome this problem. Section 4 gives disabled people the right to have an assessment of their needs for services. The NHS and Community Care Act 1990 has taken this a stage further and, under section 47(1)(a), obliges social services departments to carry out assessments:

'where it appears ... that any person for whom they may provide or arrange for the provision of community care services may be in need of any such services'.

The important distinction is that the obligation to carry out the assessment is independent of a request for one. Under the Disabled Persons Act 1986, the person must be assessed for all services under the Chronically Sick and Disabled Persons Act 1970. Under the NHS and Community Care Act 1990 the assessment can be more restricted and limited to the community services that the person seems to need. However, the Penfold judgment (January 1998) ruled that this cannot be used as a simple screening exercise but must be for all services that the local authority has power to provide and not just those that it does provide.

The Disabled Persons Act, for the first time in legislation, considers the needs of carers. Section 8(1) states that when:

(a) a disabled person is living at home and receiving a substantial amount of care on a regular basis from another person (who is not a person employed to provide such care by anybody in the exercise of its functions under any enactment) and,

(b) it falls to a local authority to decide whether the disabled person's needs call for the provision by them of any services for him under any of the welfare enactments, the local authority shall, in deciding that question, have regard to the ability of that person to continue to provide such care on a regular basis.

The right of a carer to an assessment under the Carers (Recognition and Services) Act 1995 can be contrasted with the situation under the Disabled Persons Act, which simply requires the social services department to 'have regard to' the carer's ability to provide care.

The Carers Act

The Carers (Recognition and Services) Act 1995 – 'Carers Act' for short – gives some legal recognition of the work that carers do. Under the Act, a carer who provides (or intends to provide) substantial care on a regular basis is entitled to an assessment, if requested, when a local authority social services department carries out an assessment (or re-assessment) of a person being cared for in respect of community care services (under section 47(1)(a) of the National Health Service and Community Care Act 1990) or services for children (for the purpose of the Children Act 1989 or section 2 of the Chronically Sick and Disabled Persons Act 1970). The result of the carer's assessment must be taken into consideration when the local authority is making decisions about services to be provided to a service user.

The terms 'regular' and 'substantial' are subjective, and each case is decided on its own merit and common sense. Three hours of care a week may be substantial for some carers, especially if they are working or have another family to look after.

In the lead-up to the implementation of the Carers Act in 1996, the Department of Health published Policy Guidance and a Practice Guide. The Policy Guidance sets out the government's view of *what* local authorities should do to implement the Act, and the Practice Guide gives advice on *how* it might be implemented. (Both are available from the Department of Health, address on p 112.)

The principles of the Carers Act apply throughout England, Wales, Scotland and Northern Ireland. The legislation applies fully only to England and Wales.

In Scotland all carers of adults have the right, under the Carers Act, to request an assessment from their social work department. However, it is the Children (Scotland) Act that, since April 1997, gives rights to parents and can require a local authority to provide additional services to young carers.

In Northern Ireland, the Department of Health and Personal Social Security has issued guidance to Health and Social Services Trusts, stating that all carers should be offered an assessment, and that this should be taken into account when determining what care services to provide.

The success of the Carers Act depends largely on the ability of the professional workers to find ways to meet the needs identified in a carer's assessment. This is particularly important because there are no additional resources for local authorities to undertake assessments or provide extra services. Professionals working with carers need to be creative and original, and to have a good knowledge of the existing resources available from a variety of organisations and agents.

'I knew about the carers' assessment, but I didn't see the point of asking for one because it didn't mean I would definitely get extra help.' A carer on the subject of the Carers Act

The Act is a framework or 'tool' that highlights the situation of carers and encourages people to think of ways to provide more support. However, a tool is effective only when operated correctly. The following are some basic principles that professionals working with carers should consider.

ALL CARERS SHOULD BE INFORMED OF THEIR POSSIBLE RIGHT TO REQUEST A SEPARATE ASSESSMENT

Many carers will not know about the Carers Act, and it is not enough just to ask how the carer is managing. Carers should be told of their right, and how they may get an assessment for themselves.

THE PERSON GIVING THE ASSESSMENT SHOULD ENSURE THAT THE CARER UNDERSTANDS WHAT 'ASSESSMENT' MEANS

Some carers may be confused by the term 'assessment' because of their experience of assessments being carried out to establish the financial situation of the person they are caring for and that person's ability to pay for services.

Young carers, particularly if they are at school, may relate the word to a test to see how they are doing, rather than to see if they can get more help.

CARERS SHOULD BE FULLY INVOLVED IN THE ASSESSMENT

Carers must feel able to participate fully in the assessment process. This means giving them the choice of where and when the assessment will take place; making sure they know what will happen during the assessment; and encouraging them to include as much detail as possible about any difficulties they are experiencing. The carer's own history and expertise should also be recognised and respected.

THE RIGHTS OF THE CARED-FOR PERSON MUST BE MAINTAINED

The carer's assessment gives the carer an opportunity to speak freely about their own feelings and needs. It is not, however, designed to help the carer impose their will on the person they are caring for. At times, conflict and tension exist between the carer and the person cared for, but these should be seen as a normal part of caring. The skill of the professional should help people to deal with those conflicts.

Principles such as these should raise some questions for you.

- How can you ensure that carers get the right information, in the right way and at the right time?
- Who should do the assessments if there is a conflict of interest between the carer and the person they are caring for?
- How can a need identified in an assessment be met if there are too few resources?

These questions are discussed in this handbook. It does not offer a total solution but provides ideas and a base on which to build.

Who is entitled to a carer's assessment?

The Carers Act says that a carer is entitled to an assessment if:

- they are in a caring situation, or intend to be in the near future (eg if a relative is about to be discharged from hospital); *and*
- they are or will be providing a substantial amount of care on a regular basis; *and*
- the person they are caring for is also receiving an assessment or re-assessment.

It also covers young carers under the age of 18 and carers of disabled children, whether or not they are the parents.

A carer does not have to be living with the person they are caring for in order to ask for an assessment. However, the legislation does not specify what constitutes 'substantial care' or 'a regular basis', and these aspects are open to interpretation by the local authority concerned.

Who is not entitled to a carer's assessment?

A carer's assessment is not available to the following people.

- People who are employed to provide care, such as paid care assistants and district nurses.
- People who volunteer through a voluntary organisation such as Community Service Volunteers (CSV).
- Carers who are not considered to be providing a substantial amount of care on a regular basis.

KEY POINTS

- Do not assume that carers know about the Carers Act. Many will not know about their right to an assessment.
- The carer's assessment should be a joint activity that involves the carer fully.
- The carer's assessment is not designed to favour one person's needs over another's.
- The interests and rights of the person being cared for must also be maintained.

References

Better Tomorrows? by Norman Warner, commissioned and published by Carers National Association, London, 1995

Carers (Recognition and Services) Act 1995 Policy Guidance, published by the Department of Health, London, 1996

Carers (Recognition and Services) Act 1995 Practice Guide, published by the Department of Health, London, 1996

Community Care: Agenda for action. Report to the Secretary of State for Social Services by Roy Griffiths, published by HMSO, London, 1988

Speak Up, Speak Out: research amongst members of Carers National Association, published by Carers National Association, London, 1992

Still Battling? The Carers Act one year on, published by Carers National Association, London, 1997

The True Cost of Caring: A survey of carers' lost income, published by the Caring Costs Alliance, London, 1996

2 Carrying out an assessment

People who work with carers should introduce the idea of requesting an assessment for carers during their visit to a service user or patient if they can see there is a need. All of the following situations should prompt the professional to remind a carer of their rights under the Carers Act.

- A carer is feeling less able to cope, and has been advised by another professional such as a doctor to contact social services.
- A service user or patient is about to have an assessment of their needs.
- A service user or patient needs a re-assessment because their condition has changed; for example, their health has deteriorated or they are becoming less mobile.
- A patient is about to be discharged from hospital and a carer intends to look after them.

Service users at home

If you are asked to visit someone at home for the first time, it is unlikely that you will undertake an assessment then. You will need to get a feel for the situation and understand the expectations of both the carer and the service user.

Remember that a carer can request an assessment for themselves *only* if the person they are looking after is having one. (This is simply the law. In practice, some local authorities undertake direct assessments, and the National Carers Strategy (see p 67) indicates that legislation to give carers a stand-alone right to an assessment is being considered.) This may pose a problem for the carer. For example, you may find that someone who is already a service user will not request a re-assessment if they feel that their husband, wife, etc, is providing the additional help they need, even if their health or ability is deteriorating. It is understandable that help given by a competent carer who is well known might be far more preferable to that provided by an unknown person.

In a situation like this you should be alert to signs of stress or fatigue in the carer. Try to develop the skill of drawing out information during the general conversation. Comments on how lovely the garden is or how pleasant the room you are sitting in may prompt a response by the carer such as 'Doing the gardening is my relaxation, but I rarely get enough time now' or 'It could do with spring cleaning but I'm just too tired these days'.

Remember that asking appropriate questions with genuine interest may elicit the information needed to understand how a carer is really feeling. It is not about asking trick questions that do not relate to the topic of the conversation. This will only give the impression that you are being 'nosy', and will lose the confidence of both the carer and the person being cared for.

CASE STUDY

Mrs Cook has been caring for her husband since his stroke seven years ago. Both are in their late 60s. In recent months Mr Cook's condition has deteriorated. Mrs Cook has found it increasingly difficult to get her husband up in the mornings. It takes almost two hours to wash, shave and dress him. She has the beginning of arthritis in her hands and she has found that, by breakfast time, she cannot carry the hot teapot or dishes very easily. Mr Cook likes to rise at 6am. Mrs Cook has found that she is becoming more short-tempered with her husband, which then makes her feel guilty.

Social services have been providing some help in the home to enable Mrs Cook to do the shopping once a week. The Cooks are paying for this service. Care manager Clare Rudd has arranged to visit them to see if they are happy with the service.

Over a cup of tea in the conservatory, Clare asks how Mr Cook is doing. He replies that he is doing fine. Mrs Cook adds that the doctor has increased his medication and that he does tend to struggle a bit more, especially in the mornings. She goes on to explain the length of time everything takes, and that it tires her a little.

Clare explains that it might be possible to get someone in during the morning to help Mr Cook get up. However, this would not be until 8am because there are no care assistants who can start earlier than that. She suggests that perhaps they could have breakfast first and Mr Cook could have his wash and shave later.

Mrs Cook seems keen on this idea, but Mr Cook says he is unhappy about sitting around in his pyjamas for so long, and about some unknown person providing this personal service. Mrs Cook says that perhaps he is right and that they will manage.

Clare says that they should let her know if they change their minds, thanks them for the cup of tea, and leaves.

This case study is typical of the situation many carers find themselves in. They may see an offer of help as imposing something on the person they care for to make life easier for themselves. Of course, if dealt with sensitively and wisely by the care manager, life might be made easier for both of them.

Mrs Cook tried to let Clare know that she was having difficulties, but when her husband expressed his reluctance, she quickly withdrew. Clare saw this conflict as something to be left for now, perhaps because it was Mr Cook who was actually her service user and, on the face of it, things didn't seem too bad.

It may be that Mrs Cook would want to continue caring for her husband for as long as possible. However, assumptions should not be made. A number of points need to be considered when a care manager finds a situation such as this.

- Do not assume that the carer is willing to continue caring.
- The environment in which you spend 20–30 minutes with a service user and their carer may not reflect the tensions being experienced through the day.
- Advance information about their entitlement to assessment, either by letter to the carer or, if possible, by a telephone call, may encourage the carer to ask for an assessment in private.
- Do not assume that you already know a lot about the carer; there may be much more that you don't know.
- Carers often have great difficulty in saying 'no'.

How the meeting between Clare and Mr and Mrs Cook could have ended

Clare tells Mr and Mrs Cook that she realises the service she has suggested might not be acceptable, and that she will try to think of how else they could be helped.

She has the opportunity of a few words alone with Mrs Cook as they both walk to the front door. She hands Mrs Cook some information about assessments for carers, and tells her that, if she wants to talk in private, it can be arranged. Although there may not be a perfect answer, just talking about the difficulties would be a start.

Service users in hospital

If you are working with someone who is about to be discharged from hospital, the assessments should be undertaken *before* the discharge. This is because there may be a need for essential items such as lifting equipment for bathing, or adaptations for mobility in the home. Making arrangements such as these takes time, so you should discuss assessments as soon as possible after someone is admitted into hospital. There is also the possibility that the patient will receive continuing health care services from the NHS after being discharged from hospital. If it is decided that certain services will be provided at home, a timetable must be agreed for their commencement.

KEY POINTS

- Carers should be reminded of the Carers Act and encouraged to take up their right to an assessment by caring professionals.
- If a service user or patient chooses not to have an assessment or a re-assessment of their needs, the carer cannot ask for an assessment for themselves.
- If someone has been admitted to hospital, you should be talking with them and their carer about the assessment procedure as soon as possible, *before* discharge from hospital.
- The health service may provide care or services (eg continence advice or supplies) after discharge from hospital.

The assessment

Setting the scene

Once a carer has requested an assessment of their own, they will want to know when, where and how it will be done. Where it is done should be the carer's choice. They may choose to have the assessment in their own home, in the lounge or the garden, or elsewhere such as a social services office. It should be wherever the carer feels most comfortable and able to talk easily. If the carer prefers to have the assessment away from home, alternative care may have to be arranged.

The assessment must be done when the carer has enough time. Worrying about getting back to her husband or his daughter may pressure the carer into getting through the assessment quickly. As a result, some important information may be missed.

Ideally, it should also be undertaken when the person doing the assessment has enough time. Carers are aware of the pressure most professionals are under. If you are having to look at your watch every ten minutes, they will lose confidence and try to hurry through it for you.

It may be helpful for the carer to have a practice self-assessment form some time before the actual assessment. This will give them more time to think about it. It will also enable them to focus on their role as a carer, the main difficulties they experience and what they would find helpful. A practice assessment produced by Carers National Association is given on pages 29 and 30.

Various models of assessment

There is no standard or universal model of assessment. Across the UK, local authorities have, or are in the process of developing further, their own standards and procedures. Here we identify some good examples of what should be included in an assessment for carers and the different ways in which assessments can take place.

You may find that some carers regard the assessment as some kind of test that they must pass, and try to give what they think are the 'right' answers. Others might feel that the assessment process makes them appear to be 'moaning' about their situation. It is important to reassure them that neither of these is the case, and there are exercises such as the practice self-assessment or keeping a diary that, with reassurance from the care professional, will help carers to understand this.

> 'There are so many other carers who have to do much more than me. I shouldn't complain really.' Carer of her disabled father, as well as mother of three children under the age of 10

Some social services departments have developed a brief form for carers to use to help them get ready for an assessment. Suggesting topics likely to be covered and questions to think about help to remind carers of what they would like to say during the assessment. Working through a practice assessment will prepare the carer for the 'real thing', and help them to get more out of it. It will also help them to realise just how much care they are providing.

Practice carer's assessment form

On pages 29 and 30 is a self-assessment form taken from *How do I get help: a carer's guide to assessments*, produced by the Carers National Association and printed here with their permission. It demonstrates the topics and questions that should be covered in the assessment undertaken by the social services department. (**Please note** that there would normally be space after each question for carers to write their answers.)

Another way of helping carers to recognise the level of care they provide, and to decide what sort of help they might need, is to suggest that they keep a diary of what they do over a period of time. Although this is yet another task for the carer, it really will help them to realise how much they do, and will help you to focus on the important issues. Keeping a diary might also help the carer identify the tasks that they cannot do, as well as what help they feel is needed.

You can help reduce the effort needed to record the events of one week by providing a simple record sheet for the carer to fill in. An example is given on pages 31–32 of what a completed record sheet might look like, and the sorts of things it could reveal.

Remember that this is the carer's record to help them focus on their own particular needs. They are under no obligation to share this information, but should be encouraged to do so. They may wish to use the record as a prompt for what they want you to know. This is why it is also important for you to be observant and able to interpret the full situation.

'Keeping a diary of everything we did was time-consuming, but I'm glad I did it because it made me realise how little time I have for myself.' Mother of a 30-year-old disabled woman

When it comes to filling out the official assessment form, a diary such as this will provide many indications of how the carer is coping. Before reading on, it would be a good exercise for you to read through the diary (again) and write down anything you think it is important to note.

Housing

Do you and the person you care for live together or apart? Is this arrangement satisfactory? If it is not satisfactory, say why.

Does the person you care for have any difficulty moving about in the home? (For example, climbing steps, having a bath?) If special equipment would make life easier for the person you look after, things would be easier for you.

Health

Does the person you care for have any health problems that you find hard to deal with? Describe these as fully as possible.

Do you have any health problems? If so, describe them as fully as possible. (For example, if you have a bad back, you may be able to get lifting equipment.)

Do you feel that you are getting enough sleep?

Do you feel you are suffering from stress or depression?

Time

How many hours a week do you care? Include the time you spend with the person you care for and time you spend doing other things for them such as washing, cleaning and cooking. (List the jobs you do and how long it takes you – it may surprise you!)

Do you have to help with:

- housework?
- shopping?
- bathing?
- toileting?
- other personal care (eg dressing)?
- keeping an eye on them?
- dealing with money (cashing pensions etc)?
- laundry?

Do you have to help during the day, or night, or both?

Does anyone else help with these? If so, who and for how long?

Would you like some help (or some extra help) with these jobs?

If you could have help with only one task, which would it be?

If that task was taken care of, what would be the next task you want help with? (This is to help you draw up your own list of priorities.)

Are there things you find enjoyable and relaxing that you cannot do because of your caring responsibilities? (For example, you may have given up a hobby or you may not be able to visit friends.)

When was the last time you had a whole day to yourself to do as you pleased?

Feelings

Do you feel that you don't have a choice about providing care? (You may feel that you are unable to carry on at all or only if you reduce the amount that you do. Tell the social worker about these feelings.)

What would you most like to change about your own situation?

By the time you get to this point in your practice assessment, you should have a clearer idea of what your needs and priorities are. Now go on to look at what sorts of services you might want to discuss with the social worker.

Things to discuss with the social workers

What would be helpful?

- Changes to the home and equipment to help you or the person you are caring for?
- Someone to help with personal care (eg bathing, dressing)?
- A meal delivered to the person you care for?
- Someone to help with shopping?
- A few hours' break regularly?
- A break of a week or two occasionally?
- To talk about permanent residential care?
- Counselling/talking to someone?
- To be in touch with other carers?
- Information about what is available and the costs?

	MORNING	AFTERNOON	EVENING	NIGHT
MONDAY	Got up at 6am to prepare Dad for day centre at 10.30. He was waiting around until 11.30 for the bus to arrive.	Washing machine broke down. Had to get to the laundrette before Dad came back. Too late to get it dry.	Should have visited friend, but Dad not too good. Unfair to leave him with neighbour.	Dad woke 5 times.
TUESDAY	Had a lie-in till 7 as Dad was also exhausted. Then realised we had a doctor's appointment at 10am. Almost missed it.	Laundry piling up as machine can't be fixed till tomorrow. Unable to get to laundrette with Dad. Had a visit from chiropodist.	Dad went to bed early, enabling me to get some cleaning done. Got to bed at midnight.	Dad woke 3 times.
WEDNESDAY	Up at 6 again because the washing machine is being fixed at 9. Dad being difficult.	Having my hair done at 3. Sitter came on time. Nice to have a break.	Dad seems to be coming down with a cold. Won't eat his dinner.	Very bad night. We were up for most of it.
THURSDAY	Dad quite poorly with cold. Cancelled day centre; called doctor, who came at 11.	Dad very quiet in bed. Could do with a sleep myself, but too much housework to do.	Went to bed very early. Medicine making Dad sleep heavily.	First unbroken night for 2 weeks

	MORNING	AFTERNOON	EVENING	NIGHT
FRIDAY	Dad stayed in bed till 9. Sitter came while I did the week's shopping.	Traffic jam and queues at the supermarket made me late back. Sitter very understanding, but now she would be running late.	Finally caught up with laundry. Might not have to do any over the weekend.	Dad woke twice.
SATURDAY	Up at 5.30. Dad a bit better, but now I think I have the cold.	Friend visited me, but I didn't have much time as Dad was wandering and restless.	Friend decided to stay for tea. A chance for me to have a proper conversation with someone.	Dad woke twice.
SUNDAY	Would have liked to have gone to church but couldn't get ready in time.	Cold really holding me back. Had to leave the ironing. Dad needing extra attention.	Neighbour kindly mowed our lawn. Stayed for a cup of tea.	Dad woke 3 times.

The following are points you may have picked up from the diary exercise. The carer:

- rarely has a night of unbroken sleep, and has to rise very early;
- misses company and enjoyable conversation (social isolation);
- forgoes her own needs and pleasures to look after her father;
- always has to work to a tight schedule around her father's needs;
- values the brief respite she receives to have her hair done and do the shopping;
- has a neighbour who is willing to help from time to time;
- struggles to maintain contact with her friends.

Over all, this carer could be in danger of suffering ill-health due to stress and fatigue unless she receives more support. It is worth emphasising that the assessor should not conclude that a person does not need help because the carer is providing it. It should be recorded that the person has a need and note the carer's contribution on the care plan as a service meeting this need. Otherwise, the carer's contribution is not recognised and the extent to which the person is at risk, for example if the carer is ill, may be missed.

However, in recognising these problems, the assessor could be in danger of raising the carer's expectations and then being unable to fulfil them completely. Such a situation is dealt with on pages 46–49.

Writing down the assessment

A time and place for doing the assessment should be agreed between the carer and the assessor. Not all carers will want a separate assessment, even though the Carers Act states that this is their right. Many will choose to take an assessment alongside the person they are caring for. However, it is important that it is *their* choice, and not for the convenience of the person doing the assessment or the person being cared for.

Assessment forms vary across the UK, but there should be accompanying guidance from the social services department to help the assessor ensure that the assessment is undertaken correctly and that nothing is missed out.

If your department does not have any guidance, you may find it useful to write some notes of your own beforehand. These will help you to be methodical and professional in your approach. Eventually, when you have carried out enough assessments, you will have less need for notes. Here are a few suggestions for your own guidance notes.

1 Ask if the carer is happy to have the assessment now. Are they ready?

2 Explain that you will be asking the questions set out on the assessment form and writing down, in full, the answers given by the carer. Explain that all of this will be in total confidence.

3 Explain that, once all the questions have been answered and comments made, you will repeat to them what has been said and written down.

4 Let the carer know that they can change anything they wish on the completed form.

5 Explain what will be the next step after completing the form.

6 Explain that resources are limited, and this may restrict what can be offered.

7 Keep everything simple and relaxed.

8 Be aware of your own body language. Keep your posture relaxed and open, and show that you are interested.

9 Also be aware of the carer's body language; for example, folded arms can indicate defensiveness or tension.

10 *Listen!* Always avoid the temptation to talk or interrupt the carer. Do not be tempted to give your personal opinion. (A personal opinion is different from professional experience and knowledge.)

11 Do not be over-sympathetic, or you risk seeming to be patronising. Respond appropriately and sensitively without giving the 'poor you' approach.

12 Ask the carer if there is anything else they would like to add or any areas that the form has not addressed.

It may be useful to note how long it takes to do a carer's assessment. Although most assessments will take about the same amount of time, you will find that this can vary greatly from carer to carer. A lot will depend on how the assessment is conducted; for example, you may find yourself drawn into a lengthy conversation about one aspect of caring recorded in the assessment or the carer may need to be given a lot of information. Therefore, you will need to be disciplined but diplomatic about keeping to the questions set out in the assessment.

You must make sure that you have information that is correct and relevant. Some carers may be reluctant to provide a mass of details. In these cases, you must ask yourself if you feel you have enough information, and, if not, try to get the carer to expand on their answers. Other carers may be quite the opposite, and you may have to be tactful but firm to keep the discussion on track while still enabling them to tell you all the things they think are relevant.

It is important to write down the answers clearly and in full. Writing hurried abbreviations may prove difficult to decipher later. It also means having to perform the same task again back at the office by re-writing the assessment and using valuable time unnecessarily.

Make sure that the carer has a copy of the completed assessment form. This may be given to them straight away if a carbon copy is available; otherwise, a photocopy should be sent – preferably on the same day. If your local authority's practice is to ask the carer to sign the assessment to show agreement, make sure the carer knows and feels able to refuse to sign if they disagree with the contents. It is important that you are clear about what the signature means. Some authorities require a signature to confirm that the carer has seen the assessment, not to say that they agree with it.

CASE STUDY

Care manager **Elizabeth Craig** was having a bad week. The car had broken down three times, her 8-year-old daughter had been off school with a cold (which Elizabeth was now coming down with) and she had been given five cases to add to her already overloaded work schedule. She was on her way to a carer's assessment, and already 20 minutes late. This delay would stack up and make her late throughout the day unless she could make sure this visit was short.

When she arrived, the carer to be assessed offered her a cup of tea, but Elizabeth explained that there wasn't much time to make tea, and suggested that they get started right away.

The assessment seemed to go fairly well as far as Elizabeth could tell. The questions were answered quickly, and they worked through the form swiftly. To help speed things up, Elizabeth used some shorthand and abbreviations.

With the assessment out of the way, Elizabeth thanked the carer. She had forgotten her diary so she said that she would phone that afternoon to arrange another visit; she added that a copy of this assessment would be with the carer within five working days. As she left, and was almost at her car, Elizabeth remembered that she should have given the carer some details about a local support group. 'Well, I can do that on the phone, too,' she thought. 'At least I have managed to gain ten minutes and won't be so late for my next client.'

Later that week, Elizabeth sat for two hours at her desk, trying to decipher some of the words she had written during the hurried assessment. Then a feeling of horror came over her as she realised she had failed to phone the carer to arrange a visit and to give her the details of the support group.

The assessment took far longer to type up than Elizabeth had expected, and it was sent to the carer three weeks later. There were a number of mistakes and misinterpretations, and the carer was not impressed.

If only Elizabeth didn't have so much to do.

This case study is fictitious but there are many elements that will ring true for most care managers – mechanical problems, family commitments, personal health concerns and a heavy workload are part of normal life, but they do get in the way of the ideal.

KEY POINTS

- A practice self-assessment and/or a record of what the carer does over a period will help the carer focus on the things they need to discuss.
- Use guidance notes to help you conduct a professional, methodical and useful assessment.
- Write the assessment clearly and in full to save time later and to make sure the record is accurate. Avoid using abbreviations.
- Make sure that the carer has a copy of the assessment as soon as possible.

Acting on the assessment

Although the Carers Act gives carers the right to an assessment, the law does not oblige local authorities to provide any additional services to carers. Indeed, local authorities currently cannot provide services direct to carers. So how do you avoid an assessment providing nothing more than a 'wish list'?

- Study the completed assessment carefully.
- Draw out the strengths and positive aspects of the assessment.
- Ensure that the carer has relevant information on sources of help.

If the assessment reveals that the carer is in need of additional support, this might not be costly. It requires the assessor/care manager to be knowledgeable and informed about local services, and to be creative and flexible in their thinking. Bear in mind that, by supporting a carer, you are also helping the person being cared for.

First of all, focus on the existing networks the carer may already have. How helpful or involved are family and friends? Next, are you fully aware of all the local voluntary organisations and what services they provide? Remember that many carers do not expect something for nothing. There may be a service available from a local voluntary organisation for a small charge that the carer is willing to pay.

The assessment may reveal something as straightforward as the carer needing someone to talk to. If you know of local counselling services and local carers' support groups that the carer can be put in touch with, there is at least something you can action on the results of the assessment, no matter how small it may seem. In many cases, a little help like this can make a major difference in the carer's life.

Extra resources

There will also be times when the assessment identifies the need for extra resources for the person being cared for; for example, lifting equipment, ramps or other ways to improve mobility in the home. This in turn will make life easier for the carer, or at least help them to prevent back problems in the future.

Not everything that can help carers has to cost money. One of the main problems that carers complain of is the overwhelming feeling of tiredness. Encouraging carers to realise that this is something that can be helped is the first step towards dealing with the problem. It may be useful to consider the sleep pattern of the person they are caring for. Is it possible to rearrange the carer's sleeping pattern to fit in more with the person they are caring for? If, for example, the cared-for person wanders at night and wants to chat but naps in the early afternoon, encourage the carer to take this opportunity to have a nap as well.

If carers cannot get to sleep when they go to bed because of all the stress and worry on their mind, suggest that they try going to bed later. This may seem strange, but there is little point in going to bed simply to lie there wide awake, tossing and turning with frustration at not being able to fall asleep. Indeed, research suggests that getting into a state at this time merely makes the problem worse. Reading a novel or doing something to distract the mind or having a long relaxing bath may help.

Relaxation

Another possibility is to learn relaxation techniques, which can also be beneficial in reducing stress. Many local authorities offer evening classes in yoga, aromatherapy, stress reduction and so on. In Northern Ireland carers can get information from the Educational Guidance Service for Adults.

For people who think this sort of approach is too unfocused, why not suggest exercise or sport. This can help, because it relaxes taut muscles and causes the body to relax afterwards. Being fitter can also help with the physical demands of being a carer. Details of beginners' classes and clubs should be available through the local authority.

If carers cannot get out to attend classes, there are some things that can be done at home. For example, slow gentle breathing can induce a state of relaxation. It is not quite as easy as it sounds and needs to be practised to become effective but encouraging carers to follow the four steps listed below can be helpful.

1 Sit comfortably or lie on the floor (or in bed or in the bath if that is the only time you get to yourself).
2 Breathe in, count one, let your breath out.
3 Now breathe in, count one, two, and breathe out counting one, two.
4 Keep going slowly and regularly until you get to five. The aim is to let your mind go blank of anything but the deep regular breathing. Saying the numbers is to stop your brain thinking of other things, such as the doctor's appointment the next day.

Counselling

Carers often want someone to talk to outside the family, who can help them through a difficult period in their lives, but they may feel guilty about this. You can be supportive by helping them to recognise their feelings and identify the need for counselling without seeing this as a failing.

HOW TO FIND A COUNSELLOR

National Health Service GPs can refer someone for counselling through the NHS, but they may first need to be convinced that the carer is having serious difficulties that are affecting their health.

Voluntary and charitable agencies Many groups offer counselling. Often this is free or a donation may be requested. The local Citizens Advice Bureau should be able to advise on what is available in the area.

Referring to the Samaritans may also be helpful. Sometimes carers reach a point where all they need is someone to talk to, someone to let off steam to. The Samaritans are available 24 hours a day and can offer support to carers who are feeling despairing. Make sure that carers understand that you do not need to be on the verge of suicide to contact the Samaritans, or they might get the impression that you think they are unstable or at risk.

Paid counsellors The British Association for Counselling can provide lists of local member counsellors who are willing to enter into private, fee-paying arrangements.

Budgets and priorities

'I never thought when I finished my training that I would end up haggling on the telephone with providers or arguing with my boss about whether the cost of a service was really justified. I wanted to help people, not argue over money.' Social care manager

Under community care legislation, decisions about what care services to provide were to be made according to the need of the person concerned, regardless of the availability of resources. However, the amount of resources available has always played a part, and in recent years a growing number of court judgments and rulings have challenged the law. Two examples are the Gloucestershire and the Sefton rulings. In Gloucestershire the local authority argued successfully that resources available as well as a person's need should be taken into account. This relates only to the setting of eligibility criteria in relation to services for people with disabilities (under section 2 of the Chronically Sick and Disabled Persons Act 1970): once they have assessed need and agreed that the person meets their criteria, they have a duty to provide care – but the duty is to the person being cared for, not the carer. Sefton Council argued that it should be able to withhold contributions for residential and nursing home care for people whom the local authority considered to have enough savings to pay for themselves. That is, the Council failed to follow the mandatory means-test and decided to set much lower capital limits above which it would not help fund care.

Because of limited resources or funding for local authorities and a growing population of people needing services, such challenges are likely to become more common. It is important for you to consider the following key questions when discussing possible provision with the service user and their carer and before finalising a care plan.

- Are you well informed about eligibility criteria?
- Which needs meet the eligibility criteria?
- How much flexibility are you allowed in buying services?
- Are you well informed about policies and procedures that determine the maximum weekly costs of care packages? Do you need special authorisation to spend above a certain weekly level?
- Will the budget holder automatically approve certain needs but not others?
- What type of budgetary control can/should you use?
- Have you enough information to compare the cost and quality of different providers/services?
- Does the service user require the service on a long-term basis? Is the user's condition likely to remain the same, get worse or get better?
- What will the cost be to the service user? Is the user able/willing to pay the charges for the different options you are considering? Has the user's eligibility for welfare benefits been checked?
- If the cost of the package is likely to be high, does the service user qualify for help from the Independent Living Fund?
- Are you well informed about any other special budgets that you may be able to draw on for certain kinds of needs?
- Have you taken into account any health or housing services that other agencies will be providing?

Practice varies widely. Some authorities impose a cash limit on care packages for people living at home. They may require that a person whose care costs more than a cost-ceiling move into residential care if it would meet that individual's needs, including psychological needs. However, if residential care is not found to be appropriate, the local authority might have to exceed their ceiling. At present, other authorities are moving in this direction but do not formally impose a limit. You will need to be well informed and up to date about available budgets, eligibility criteria and the charging policy for care at home in your area. (See Appendix 1 for the national charging procedures that local authorities must follow for residential and nursing home care.)

There is due to be (at the time of writing) a Government initiative that will bring about greater national consistency in access to services: 'Fair Access to Care Services'.

Helping service users to make the best of their money

When a decision has been made about the services needed, a financial assessment will be undertaken. You may know from experience that going through the financial assessment forms with service users can be complicated and time-consuming. It is not surprising that charging policies and means-testing can be difficult aspects of community care: financial assessment and its result often arouse strong feelings in both users and carers.

Financial assessment can be made more productive for you, your service users and their carers if you regard it as an opportunity to explain the local authority's charging policies and procedures, and to explore users' and carers' financial situations and possible sources of financial support. You can also give them clear information about their rights and, where appropriate, tell them about independent sources of advice such as the Citizens Advice Bureau and the Carers National Association's CarersLine.

To make the best use of the time spent undertaking the financial assessment, there are six areas that you need to be well informed about. They are discussed below.

Your local authority's charging policy Carers and service users are often given contradictory or misleading information by different staff. Try to provide clear information and sort out any confusion. Carers may not like it but can at least come to terms with a charging system that they think is unfair if they understand how the system came about and that at least they are not being personally singled out but that everyone is being treated equally unfairly.

The Social Services Inspectorate Advice Note says that the person may be charged only when a service is being provided for them. So it is important to *be absolutely clear about not assessing the finances of the service user and the carer jointly.* Any charges made for domestic and day care must be reasonable for the user to pay, and they can complain if they think that the charges are unreasonable.

Anomalies in charging policy Charging policies for day care and domiciliary services vary widely. What, if any, charges are made is a matter of local authority discretion. If there are areas of dispute about whether charges are reasonable, carers and service users who are likely to be affected should be told that they have a right to appeal against the charges. Services cannot be withdrawn while an appeal is underway, but it is possible for a debt to build up if the user does not pay any charges that it is eventually decided are payable.

Health authority policy on who is eligible for NHS-funded continuing care The sort of care that might be involved here is very wide ranging: for example, special equipment, continence advice and supplies, chiropody, speech therapy, respite health care and rehabilitation. It also includes NHS continuing inpatient care, which can be provided in its own long-stay hospitals or by the NHS purchasing care in a private or voluntary sector nursing home. Health authorities must follow the guidance given in HSG(95)5, *NHS responsibilities for meeting continuing health care needs*, when drawing up their criteria to decide who will qualify for which NHS continuing health care services. If the health authority agrees that the person meets its criteria for continuing inpatient care and it funds this care in an independent sector nursing home, the person will not be charged for that care. Paying for nursing home care may be the responsibility of the health authority, and so is free to the user. In such an instance, however, the person would be treated as an NHS hospital patient, and any state benefits they have been receiving might reduce or cease over time.

If the person does not meet their health authority's criteria for NHS continuing inpatient care, they may still be assessed as needing care in an independent sector nursing home. In this case, however, they would be expected to pay towards the costs, following the national means-test system administered by the local authority. If contributions to nursing home charges are made by the local authority, these are means-tested. Policies are agreed locally but must be in line with the national guidance. You should be aware of the eligibility criteria of any health authority that you deal with. This is particularly so since the Coughlan case.

Pamela Coughlan is a woman with severe physical disabilities living in Mardon House, a purpose-built NHS nursing home in Devon. In 1998 North and East Devon Health Authority attempted to close the home and move the residents to nursing homes in the independent sector. Crucially the Coughlan case raised the issue of who is responsible for funding long-term nursing care. The health authority had assumed that, under Department of Health Guidance (HSG (95)8 *NHS responsibilities for meeting continuing healthcare needs*), it was no longer responsible for purchasing long-term nursing care. Its belief that this was now the job of social services departments was clearly reflected in the eligibility criteria it developed. These criteria stated that it would not fund 'general' nursing care, which it defined as 'including nursing observation, care and treatment which requires a nurse in constant attendance'.

Pamela Coughlan won her case in the High Court in December 1998, with the ruling that the NHS was responsible for all nursing care, regardless of where it was provided. The health authority appealed against the decision, but in July 1999 the Court of Appeal upheld it, ruling that North and East Devon Health Authority's criteria were unlawful. Although it went a long way to clarify the boundary between NHS and local authority responsibility for long-term care, it did not draw a precise legal line. The Court of Appeal made it clear that nursing care should be provided under the National Health Service Act 1977. The central part of the ruling drew on section 21 of the National Assistance Act 1948, under which local authorities have a duty to provide accommodation for certain vulnerable groups. The Appeal Court judgment stated that, under the 1948 Act, social services can provide some nursing services but only if they are 'merely incidental or ancillary' to the provision of the accommodation.

This means that the NHS can transfer responsibility for some nursing care to the local authorities but it cannot do so if a patient's primary need for accommodation is a health need — as it was in the Coughlan case. The ruling indicated that the Department of Health's guidance, on which the health authority's eligibility criteria were based, was flawed. The judgment indicates that anyone with health needs similar to or greater than those of Pamela Coughlan requires accommodation primarily because of their health needs and so is entitled to longer-term NHS nursing care.

In any case, you should refer the user to their GP or the health authority if you think that they might need NHS services, so that the NHS can take part in the assessment of the person's needs and so that any services that the NHS decides to provide or arrange are taken into account when the social services department decides what services it will offer. Similarly, if the person might need services from the housing authority, it too should be involved in the assessment.

The social services department's complaints procedure A carer or service user can ask for a review of the financial assessment through the complaints procedure if they believe that they have been wrongly assessed or unfairly charged for services. The whole area of charges, benefits, liability to pay charges for social services etc is extremely complicated. If you are not an expert, the best thing to do is to refer to agencies that are.

Welfare benefits and sources of advice Ensuring that carers and service users are making the best use of their incomes by claiming everything to which they are entitled is very important. The *Disability Rights Handbook* is an invaluable source of information and can be obtained from the Disability Alliance (address on p 113).

Grants Some carers and service users may not be aware that they could be eligible for a grant from a professional association, trade union, armed forces charity or other local grant-making charity. *A Guide to Grants for Individuals in Need* and the *Directory of Grant-making Trusts* can be found in the reference section of most local libraries. The organisation Charity Search or the Association of Charity Officers (addresses on pp 111 and 110) may be able to suggest sources of financial help for older people, as may local charity information bureaux.

Sources of independent financial advice You need to keep yourself well informed about which local agencies (eg Age Concern England or the Citizens Advice Bureau) can offer reliable benefits and financial advice.

When action is not possible

A carer's assessment often uncovers a need for help, some greater than others, and there will be times when it is not possible to provide what is needed. This is particularly the case if, for example, substantial services are already in place for the person being cared for, and are adequate for them. It should be explained very clearly to the carer why a service cannot be offered. It is at this stage that the 'care plan' is very important. The care plan is not the record of the assessment but rather it is a statement of what help the person will actually be getting — the 'package of care'. This needs to be set out clearly because people cannot challenge failure to provide services as specified unless they have a specification. The care plan should also highlight how the carer's role fits in with other services, and is a clear way of recognising the carer's input. It is not easy to give this sort of information, but carers generally appreciate honesty and should not be made promises that cannot be kept.

If a carer is unhappy about a decision following an assessment, you should first try to resolve this together. If it cannot be resolved in this way, the carer can appeal. It is the duty of the care manager to make sure that carers know about their right to appeal against any decision. It is important for them and the care manager to understand that this is not a complaint about a person, but a request to have a decision reconsidered.

Appeals procedures may vary, but will be the same for some aspects because the appeal is made via the complaints procedure. The social services department must have a designated complaints officer and must be able to give information about making a complaint. There are various time limits that must be observed, and particular requirements for the make-up of the review panel if the complaint reaches stage 3. (Stage 1 is an informal complaint; stage 2 is a formal complaint to the designated officer.)

Details about the complaints/appeals procedure should be given to the carer before an assessment is carried out.

Reasons why a carer might want to appeal against a decision include:

- The carer feels that a particular service is necessary but it is not being, and will not be, provided.
- There is a decision to levy charges for a service, or to increase charges.
- The care manager believes that there is no need for services but the carer disagrees.
- There is a long waiting list for the service.

Whether it is regarded as an 'appeal' or a 'complaint', the carer may worry about the consequences of making representations to the social services department. Carers often think that services may be affected or withdrawn or that they will be seen as troublemakers. Of course this is not the case, and carers should be reassured that this will not happen. Many local authorities state that they encourage people to use their complaints and appeals systems, as it is a way of ensuring they are providing the services that people want.

It may be necessary to seek independent support and advice for a carer who wishes to appeal. This can be found through other voluntary organisations such as an advocacy service, a carers' worker or the Citizens Advice Bureau. The care manager may provide support in making an appeal. For example, if it is an appeal about charges, the care manager can help the carer to explain why they think the charges should not be made.

An appeal should not spoil the relationship between you, the caring professional, and the carer but this will largely depend on your attitude. It will not help matters if you become defensive and take it personally. The chances are that you will see the carer's point of view and understand their reasons for appealing. Remember that in many ways this is a partnership between you, the carer and the person being cared for. Working together to resolve the difficulties will bring support and respect for all parties.

There may also be carers who do not want the only help you are able to offer. For example, if there is local carers' support group, don't assume that you can solve a carer's problems by putting them in touch with it. Not everyone wishes, or is able, to attend group meetings.

For information about what someone can do if they wish to challenge a decision or they do not like the service(s) they have been offered, see Appendix 2.

Recording unmet needs

There will be times when it is just not possible to provide the help a carer needs. Do not feel defeated because of this. If you have given it your best shot and drawn a blank, the next best thing to do is register the gap.

When a carer's needs cannot be met, a record should be kept and used as part of a feedback mechanism to local authority managers. You will need to find out what feedback mechanism exists in your authority, and your part in it. If possible, explain to the carer how this mechanism works so they can see that at least the information will be noted or reconsidered at some point.

The importance of a feedback mechanism cannot be over-stated. It is a way of identifying common problems in service provision, whether it be about a geographical area with a certain user group, the way in which resources are distributed or simply the lack of such resources.

KEY POINTS

- Not all of carers' needs are costly.
- Many carers are willing to pay a small charge for some extra help.
- Be honest and realistic about what help you are able or not able to offer.
- An appeal or complaint about the result of a carer's assessment should not be seen as a personal attack. Your skill as a professional should enable you to support carers in every way. This will strengthen the partnership in caring.
- One way of working towards more support for carers is to make sure that all the unmet needs are registered.

3 Working with other agencies

One of the keys to working with and supporting carers is knowing who else is out there. It is important to build your networks to ensure that you know about other services and people, and, just as important, that they know about you and your work. Building this kind of network has two main purposes. First, it provides you with information that can be passed on direct to carers, and, secondly, it may also provide some support for you and the work you are doing.

This chapter lists a number of types of agencies that are likely to operate in the same field of work as you, or that provide additional sources of information that may be needed by you or carers.

Make sure that you keep your information up to date. People often come and go, so it is important that you have the right contact names. Make sure that they also know about your work, and keep them informed about what you are doing. Obviously, this does not mean disclosing information about individual carers, but more about general trends and the needs of carers over all. You may have ideas you would like to share with other professionals. In recognising the valuable work done by other people, you are likely to gain their interest and support in return.

Storing this kind of information on the computer back at the office may be helpful, but it will be more beneficial if it is also stored in a notebook in your pocket, bag or briefcase. This will make the information you need available instantly at all times, and you can add to it whenever you encounter another potential supporting agency.

This chapter also explains how you and other agencies might develop a joint approach to support carers. At a time when most budgets are tight, other agencies will also be interested in working with you to develop useful and effective ways of supporting carers.

Doctors' surgeries

A variety of professional and nursing help is available via GP surgeries. They can include district nurses, continence advisers, diabetes nurses and health visitors. Make sure you have a current list of doctors' surgeries in the area you work in. You can get the list from your local health authority.

District nurses make home visits to give skilled nursing care and treatment. They can also give advice on concerns such as lifting and the management of medication, and can act as a conduit to the specialist nurses such as continence advisers or diabetes nurses.

Continence advisers can give specialist advice on coping with incontinence and how to make the problem more manageable.

Diabetes nurses educate and advise patients and carers of people with insulin- and non-insulin-dependent diabetes mellitus.

Health visitors provide health advice at home for all age groups, although they often focus on young children and babies.

Other professionals may also be contacted for help.

Dieticians give advice on nutrition and healthy eating. They provide specialist advice to professionals, patients and their carers. They may be contacted through either the GP surgery or the local hospital.

Community psychiatric nurses work with families and individuals at home or in community health settings. They are concerned with people's emotional well-being, including those with dementia. You will often hear them referred to as 'CPNs'. They can be contacted through the local hospital or the GP.

Physiotherapists are usually connected to a hospital or a health centre, but can be contacted through the GP. They are concerned with restoring or improving people's mobility after illness, an accident or an operation. All mobility aids are supplied by the hospital or community physiotherapy department via the GP. Physiotherapy is usually provided only in the short term. If a service user is prepared to pay for physiotherapy, they can contact the Chartered Society of Physiotherapy for the names of members in the area.

Occupational therapists help people to achieve or maintain independence at home, providing advice on equipment and adaptations for the home such as stair-lifts, adapted baths and toilets, and ramps. Often referred to as 'OTs', they can be contacted through hospitals, GPs' surgeries or social services. (In some parts of the UK, occupational therapists are available through all three; in others they are available only through the health service.)

Speech and language therapists are usually connected to a hospital. They provide advice and therapy for all communication disorders – ie language, speech, voice and fluency – and also on the functioning of the mouth and throat (eg swallowing food without choking).

Chiropodists can be accessed through the GP's surgery. For less complex conditions such as basic foot-care or nail-cutting, services are often provided via voluntary organisations such as Age Concern.

Community pharmacists are also health professionals who are readily available to give advice on treating common illnesses. They have detailed knowledge about medicines. Increasingly, pharmacists are maintaining computerised records of customers' medication

Some medical practices are now working closely with care workers, who can provide carers with information when they visit the surgery. However, at the time of producing this handbook, there are only a handful of such schemes in the UK. Find out from your local authority if there is one in your area: this will be an extremely useful contact to have.

Social services

The way in which local authorities operate their social services departments varies across the UK. However, there are some basic divisions that indicate areas of responsibility. Social services departments (social work departments in Scotland, or health and social services boards in Northern Ireland) are usually divided into units and teams, each being responsible for particular groups of people in the community:

- older people;
- children and families;
- people with a learning disability;
- people with a physical or sensory disability;
- people with a mental health problem;
- people with a problem of substance misuse.

There are other areas of responsibility, which may be included in the above or be separated, such as homelessness and children who are at risk. Get to know and understand how your local social services department operates, and who is responsible for what.

Some people are confused over certain jobs and job titles in social services departments. A common lack of understanding sometimes exists over the difference between, for example, 'care manager' and 'social worker'.

A *care manager* (or *team leader*) is usually someone who has a qualification in social work, occupational therapy or nursing. The original idea of 'care manager' came with the implementation of the community care reforms in 1993, when someone from social services would be responsible for putting together a complete package for a service user or patient who was ill, disabled or older/frail. The package would include any domestic help needed, meals, bathing services and respite services. The care manager would also be responsible for arranging for those services, which were usually provided by social services themselves.

Since 1993, many services are contracted out to private and voluntary organisations, sometimes called the 'independent sector'. The care manager has responsibility for booking and budgeting for such services, as well as for putting together the care package.

A *social worker*, on the other hand, is usually concerned with more specific and individual problems such as child protection, domestic violence and juvenile delinquency. Nevertheless, in many social services departments, social workers carry out the care assessments even if they don't have a budget. If they do have a budget, they are able to make care arrangements up to certain levels. (The term 'social worker' was used quite widely in the past but nowadays often describes someone with a professional (DSW or CQSW) qualification.)

Carers' projects

Over the past ten years, support for carers has increased with the development of many new ideas and projects by voluntary organisations such as the Carers National Association, the Princess Royal Trust, the Crossroads Care Attendant Schemes and Community Service Volunteers (CSV). There may be a carers project or similar scheme in your area.

Carers' projects are often funded or part-funded by the local authority. The aims of a project are to ensure that carers are:

- informed about all aspects of caring for someone;
- informed about what help is available;
- consulted on issues such as community care plans.

Carers' projects also aim to promote the interests of carers. Some may 'specialise', for example, in supporting black carers, young carers, gay and lesbian carers and carers of people with dementia. Others are more generic, providing support to all carers. The projects may also run support groups, carers' forums and other events to provide support and information for carers.

Information about carers' projects that are local to you should be available through a number of sources, including libraries, local authorities, local Age Concern groups, Citizens Advice Bureaux,

Councils for Voluntary Services (CVS) and the telephone directory. Although most carers' projects are mainly concerned with information, advocacy and support, some provide direct services such as respite care or sitting services.

People who work for carers' projects, such as carers' workers and development workers, are often keen to talk to other professionals in the health and social services in order to promote their work with carers. They are useful contacts to have, and can provide a wide variety of information relating to carers' needs and local services.

Other organisations

Although carers' projects and other such schemes are obvious resources to know about, there are other organisations that may not be directly concerned with carers but can be of great help in building up a network of carer support and information (as well as matters relating to people being cared for). The 'Useful addresses' section at the back of this book (pp 109–118) lists national organisations with useful information, many of which have branches or regional groups across the country.

Contacting the listed organisations

As organisations can move offices and change telephone numbers, the contact numbers and addresses given in the 'Useful addresses' section may become out of date. However, local libraries and telephone enquiries will provide up-to-date information on whom to contact and where.

Most large organisations can supply information packs about their work and information about the services they provide in your area. (A large stamped addressed envelope with a written request is often much appreciated.)

Make sure you know your local volunteer bureau; it can often provide volunteers to undertake tasks such as gardening and driving. Other sources of support for carers may be provided by certain religious groups, local Women's Institutes and other local associations.

Knowing of their existence and getting yourself known to them will increase your ability to find support for carers.

'It would be so helpful if I could find out what people were responsible for without having to ring round numerous departments.' A carer without a care manager

KEY POINTS

- The wider your knowledge of other sources of help and information, the greater the opportunities you will have for carer support.
- A notebook of useful contacts will give you more immediate information during your visits to carers than the computer back at the office.
- Make sure that you have a basic understanding of the roles of other people in health and social services. It will help to reduce the confusion for carers if you can explain the various responsibilities.

Developing a joint approach to supporting carers

The more you know about who else is out there, the greater will be your ability to provide support for carers. You also need to know how willing others are to develop a joint approach with you. It would be helpful if they also knew how they might benefit, apart from being seen to provide a good service to carers.

The health services and the social services should be partners working together to support carers: the Department of Health has produced guidance (*Carers (Recognition and Services) Act Policy Guidance*) for both authorities to do so. Nevertheless, other agencies need not be excluded from a joint approach. Pooling resources to provide a more comprehensive service can benefit everyone.

Promoting a multi-agency approach means that there are likely to be a number of people involved in visiting a service user or patient and their carer at home. They include advisers on housing and benefits, gardening volunteers and 'home helps', occupational therapists, chiropodists, care managers, volunteer drivers, hairdressers, district nurses, people from befriending schemes, counsellors and so on. The list could be endless and might create worry and confusion for both the carer and the person they are caring for. In this situation, it is even more important to keep carers informed of who does what.

CASE STUDY

It had taken care manager Clare Rudd four months to involve a number of other people in supporting **Miss Simpson** and her disabled older brother. Clare was pleased that the local volunteer bureau could provide someone to sit with Mr Simpson regularly so that Miss Simpson could have a break. She had also arranged for some help with shopping and cleaning, advice on adaptations in the home and a visit from a local carers' worker to give Miss Simpson some information about carers' support groups.

However, on a visit to the Simpsons, Clare discovered that things were not going as well as she thought. Miss Simpson explained that she had been promised a hand rail in the bathroom for her brother several weeks ago but had heard nothing since. Mr Simpson needed a lot of physical support and, as she was not a strong person, this was continuing to cause her concern. Miss Simpson could not remember exactly when the need for a hand rail had been agreed, or the name of the person who made the visit to assess the need.

Clare said she would follow it up for the Simpsons. They then sat down and spent the next hour filling in forms to enable Miss Simpson to claim Invalid Care Allowance.

Some weeks later Miss Simpson was informed that she had made two applications for Invalid Care Allowance. Clare discovered that, when the local carers' worker had visited Miss Simpson, she too had helped her to apply for Invalid Care Allowance, but Miss Simpson had become confused and thought she was applying for Income Support.

It was clear that, although the Simpsons were now able to get the support they needed, the number of people involved was creating confusion and often wasting time for both the visitors and the Simpsons.

Was there a way of avoiding these difficulties?

A possible solution

Even though you may build a network of support for carers, it is unrealistic to think you will always be in communication with each other over the concerns of all your service users and carers. You need to find ways of ensuring that information flows both ways for all parties.

In Worcestershire, the Elgar Housing Association's Stay-Put and Housing Advice Service has produced a booklet to enable people to keep track of who visits them and for what purpose. This *Professional and Carer Visitors Record* is divided into five short sections.

Section A explains how to use the record book and includes a page of useful telephone numbers, with space for people to add others.

Section B is a record of professionals and others who visit, which should be filled in with the following information whenever a professional worker visits:

- Name of the visitor
- Date of the visit
- Telephone number
- Job title and organisation
- Reason for the visit

Section C is a record of benefits requested:

- Which benefit has been applied for
- Who has made or helped with the application
- The date of application
- The result

Sections D and E record any alarm faults and monthly alarm tests for older and/or disabled people who have subscribed to the Stay-Put alarm system.

This method of recording is valuable for both the carer and the professional. The carer knows exactly who is visiting, and can refer to previous visits when following something up – such as the promised hand rail in the case study. For professionals such as Clare Rudd, valuable time can be saved by having all the relevant information in one place.

If no such scheme is in operation in your area, perhaps you could suggest to carers that they keep a notebook. In it they can keep a record of who visits them, when and for what purpose, which could then be shared with you or other professional visitors to the carer's home. The notebook could incorporate, for example, the care plan provided by social services: it will set out which services they are arranging and providing, and (ideally) the name of the worker(s) and who they work for, and when they will come and what job they will do.

KEY POINTS

- One of the most valuable time and money savers for carers is being able to get all the information they need from one service.
- There are many organisations that, although not directly concerned with carers, may be of considerable help in providing relevant help and information.
- Encouraging the carer to develop a simple record of visitors will help keep you up to date on how well the support is going.

Community care plans and community care charters

The input of carers into the drawing up of community care plans and community care charters is essential if these are to have any relevance for them.

The main elements of the community care plan should be:

- A focus on agreed service developments.
- Clear targets relating to these service developments.
- An overview of proposed service developments and targets for the future.

Overall targets may include:

- To co-ordinate and publish a directory of all agencies providing a community care service, enabling carers and the helping agencies to keep in touch.
- To issue leaflets to inform carers about the main services, whom they aim to help and how carers can find out more.
- To provide all information in a choice of large print, audiotape and Braille, and in different languages.
- To hold meetings throughout the year to which carers can come and comment on how service providers are doing and to hear views on how services can continue to improve.
- To select key social service areas each year for special customer care initiatives as part of a commitment to continuous improvement of services.
- To tell carers how local standards for services have been achieved, compared with national performance indicators.

The community care charter should provide:

- A short guide to the main community care services.
- What people can expect from the health and social services.
- Basic information on standards in community care.
- Performance targets for each service.
- An explanation of what service users and carers can do if their needs are not being met.

Some community care plans and charters have a separate section on carers, whereas others include carer issues in the various sections. Opinion is divided as to which is better, but we feel that *both* should be done. By adding carers to each section, the recognition of carers and carers' issues can be lost; by thinking about carers only in a discrete section risks overlooking their needs in other areas. Mentioning carers in both places ensures that carers are recognised both in their own right and in relation to why they are carers in the first place.

Long-term care charters

Better Care, Higher Standards, the framework for long-term care charters published by the Department of Health, has a section referring to carers' expectations. Local authorities will have to devise long-term care charters just as they currently do for community care services, and it is important that the principles outlined in this chapter are applied when this is done.

Consultation with carers' groups

Now that many social services departments are organised along 'user group' lines, there can be a tendency to see the interests of carers as being satisfactorily represented through existing user groups. Whilst this can be the case, carers may have needs different from or conflicting with those of the person for whom they are caring. It is important to acknowledge this fact. The establishment and rapid growth of carers' groups around the country suggests that carers themselves perceive a common interest – their own needs for support – to which local authorities should respond.

CASE STUDY

Frank has cared for his wife for the past two years, after she had a major stroke. Recently, his local carers' worker has been encouraging him to consider going to a coffee morning held by a small group of carers.

Eventually, Frank went along, and was surprised to find that it wasn't just a 'talking shop' but a lively and friendly group with lots of common interests. He learned that, as well have having coffee mornings for mutual support, the group sometimes invited guests to talk about their work or their organisation. Next week it would be a talk about benefits by someone from the local Citizens Advice Bureau.

Frank found it quite comforting that there were other people who really knew how he was feeling. Not only that, but they also shared ideas on how they managed through difficult times and even had the odd laugh about it.

Frank wished that he had known about the group sooner; during the first two years of caring for his wife, he had felt that no one understood. The group became a lifeline and respite for a few hours a week, where he not only found the support he needed but was also able to support others.

In addition to finding and giving support at the carers' group, Frank gradually was able to talk about his feelings at the carers' forum, which was a quarterly event attended by a number of groups. The forum would often invite people from health and social services, and carers could put forward their concerns and suggestions for improving services.

At last Frank felt he was able to influence the decisions that so affected him and his wife.

Where carers have been recognised as a group separate from service users, some local authorities feel that they should try to find 'representative carers'. But what are they seeking carers to represent? Like those they care for, carers differ greatly: they are young, middle-aged and elderly, live in urban, rural or suburban environments, may belong to an ethnic minority group, may be in full- or part-time paid employment, and may or may not live with the person they care for. They may be short-term or long-term carers or may no longer be caring for someone. They all have a legitimate concern for service provision. They all have something to contribute. The individual care packages acknowledge the differences that exist between people who are receiving care. The same acknowledgement of individual differences should be extended to carers.

If consultation is simply seen as a duty for the local authority and a right for carers, this persuades neither that both sides can benefit from the process. Carers need to be convinced that consultation is going to be useful to them as well as to the local authority.

Carers who belong to ethnic minorities may have distinctive problems to which particular attention should be paid. It is not that their needs as carers are necessarily different, but they may want them to be met in different ways. Some local authorities (such as Bury and Hounslow) use specialist workers to assist in consulting with minority groups in their area. This subject is discussed more fully in Chapter 5.

When setting up consultation it is important to consider who else, apart from carers and users of services, should be involved. Where consultation is well established, carers feel that it is essential for a wide range of professionals and voluntary agencies to participate in the process. In some areas it seems that the local authority has taken the lead in consulting carers and in others the health authority has been more active. The effective implementation of community care depends on the commitment and co-operation of all agencies.

How much time can you spend on consultation?

Time spent away from caring is precious. The demands of legislation and the constraints of limited finance clearly place a heavy load on those employed by local authorities to offer services. However, this responsibility is defined, time-limited (in terms of hours worked) and rewarded, and is usually shared and supported by colleagues. The task of the carer has no such limits or definitions – it stretches through days and nights and over years. There are no tangible rewards and it is frequently solitary.

The aim of consultation is to ease the burden on carers as well as making service provision more efficient. You therefore have a special duty to ensure that consultation does not waste carers' time. This is particularly the case since many carers now have experienced 'consultation fatigue' and have questioned the value of the process. How much consultation do you *need*?

In some ways it is impossible to say how much consultation is enough but it is important to consider this question if a lot of time and effort is not to be wasted. Sometimes, because of anxieties about the 'representativeness' of carers, the temptation is to attempt a vast consultation exercise. When little imagination and effort are put into this, for example where it is limited to an advertisement in the free local newspaper asking for comments, the response is likely to be disappointingly small. When a lot of effort is put in, the result can be costly, unsustainable and difficult to make use of later.

A much more satisfactory solution to the problem is for clear and permanent channels of communication to be constructed through which carers can make their views known to service providers and to other carers. Such channels can take a number of different forms:

- Carers' groups.
- Registers of carers, maintained to enable the exchange of information and to provide a readily accessible consultation audience.
- Carers' helplines, run by statutory or voluntary agencies; monitoring procedures can help in identifying emerging issues and concerns.
- Resource centres that can serve as central points of information and to collate and disseminate carers' views.
- Carers' forums – formalised, planned meetings where senior health and social services personnel can meet carers and hear their concerns.
- Progress groups of carers supported and facilitated to meet and comment on developments and issues relating to community care.

The advantages of having channels such as these are:

- Carers control how and when they express their views.
- The structures begin to influence the thinking of both carers and local authorities. Carers can be convinced that their views are genuinely sought and welcomed. Local authorities are made more aware of the carers' perspective.
- The structures begin to shape working practices. Once carers believe that their views are a valued element in planning and providing services, they will be encouraged to play a greater part in

consultation. Local authorities are more likely to be able to assimilate into practice the results of a steady flow of information than the indigestible mass that results from consultation on a grand scale.

Consultation should be a realistic process of influencing services; it should not be limited to just listening to carers. It is also important that their views be recorded and passed on to relevant departments and that carers receive feedback on what has or has not happened as a result. An example of the way this can be done is the Canterbury and Thanet Carers' Forum. A representative from the social services department attends the meeting to present the proposals in the community care plan. Having done so, he or she withdraws to allow carers to discuss this among themselves. Points that are raised are recorded by the carers' worker, who also acts as the facilitator. When the social services representative returns, each point is dealt with in turn and a record kept of the response. Carers are assured that their comments will be reported back to the department and that they will receive a written response. In Hounslow and Aberdeen, carers' comments are included in the community care plan, and the Home from Home replacement care scheme in Rotherham uses questionnaires after placements to gauge the success of the service.

In practice most of the business of consulting carers takes place in meetings. For many carers these represent a real obstacle to becoming involved, as they can find them intimidating and confusing. There are a number of ways that you can make meetings more 'carer-friendly'.

- A number of authorities have recognised the value of staff attending carers' meetings as well as inviting carers to attend their meetings.
- When carers are invited to join planning groups, they can make better use of the opportunity if the terms of reference and the purpose of the meetings are made clear to them beforehand. Plenty of notice of meetings should be given, and paperwork kept to a minimum.

■ Carers' support workers may attend meetings on behalf of carers to get a feel for what goes on and report back to carers, who may later decide that they would like to attend in future. When this happens, it is better if more than one carer can attend so that they give each other moral support. Moral support can also come from a member of staff acting as mentor to guide carers through the meeting, explaining what is unfamiliar and alerting other professionals to the need to be sensitive to the needs of carers in this situation. This is particularly important in the face of professional jargon, which many carers find a problem.

■ A practical way of helping carers deal with meetings is the briefing and de-briefing that takes place in Hounslow. Before a group of carers are involved in training sessions for professionals, the local authority's training officer explains to them the purpose of the meeting and the areas to be covered. Afterwards carers report how they felt and what they thought had been successful.

■ As well as providing a replacement care service and transport or travelling expenses, you can try to arrange meetings at times to suit carers.

■ The meeting itself should be neither too large nor too formal. In Sandwell there are photographs and descriptions of the social services personnel present and also of carers who attend regularly.

■ Above all, carers should be actively made welcome – considered rather than simply targeted. In this way they will be encouraged to see meetings as worthwhile.

A personal approach is necessary to involve carers and to keep them involved. This should include: direct invitations to attend non-threatening meetings at which carers are made to feel welcome; consideration being given to their needs for help in getting there and being made to feel comfortable when they are there; the opportunity to express their views freely; and recognition of their contribution both at the time and later, through feedback.

If all this is done there can be some hope that, in the words of a carer: 'If they listen to carers and act on what they hear, yes, consultation will make a difference'.

National Carers Strategy

The *National Carers Strategy*, published in February 1999, is an attempt to bring together measures already in place to support carers and to lay down measures to provide support, recognition and rights for carers in the future. Broadly, the strategy can be broken down into two main components representing the bringing together of existing initiatives on the one hand and new recommendations on the other.

Summary of existing initiatives

- A carer's second pension, giving carers receiving Invalid Care Allowance and Home Responsibilities Protection a credit towards a second-tier pension.
- A review of Invalid Care Allowance.
- Financial support for working carers to be kept under review.
- A grant of £750 million to local authorities in England towards rehabilitation and prevention.
- Development of family-friendly employment practices.
- Guidance on young carers and schools.
- Measures to improve the quality of services for disabled children.

Summary of new recommendations

- A new grant of £140 million to local authorities in England to help carers take a break.
- A reduction in council tax for disabled people and carers living in Band A properties.
- The possibility of extending the New Deal to help carers return to work.
- A question on carers in the census.
- More carer-friendly employment developments, with the Government taking the lead.
- New recommendations for supporting young carers.
- A future power to allow local authorities to provide services direct to carers.
- More flexibility for carers in organising their own support.
- New quality measures for local carers' centres and projects.

The development of the National Carers Strategy was a UK-wide activity involving specific consultation in Wales, Northern Ireland and Scotland. The new funding, however, is for England only. It will be the responsibility of the relevant assemblies and the Scottish Parliament to determine this in their areas.

The strategy will take time to be implemented but should help to ensure that carers' issues are kept at the top of health and social services agendas.

Putting together a carers' support strategy

The Carers' Code, produced by Carers National Association, comprises eight key principles for policy makers and service providers:

- *Recognition* of carers and of their skills and needs.
- *Choice* about whether or not the carer is able or willing to take on or continue the caring role and how to provide that care.
- *Equal access* to support and services for carers of any gender, race, culture, disability, age and sexual orientation.
- *Consultation* with carers through regular, formal and informal channels by those who provide support and services.
- *Information* that is accurate and comprehensive, provided to all carers when needed before, during and after caring.
- *Practical help*, including accessible assessment procedures and carer-focused, flexible services.
- *Maximum income* through help to claim benefits and minimum charges for carers.
- *Co-ordinated services* by all agencies working together efficiently and effectively under community care legislation.

The Carers' Code highlights the major areas that need to be considered when developing a carers' support strategy. In 1995 the Social Services Inspectorate produced two reports based on studies of local authority services for carers. *Caring Today* reflects the national inspection of local authority support to carers and *What Next for Carers?* is a report of a joint development project. (They are available from the Department of Health.)

In summary, both reports found a great deal of activity and many good examples of successful work. They also uncovered areas of work with carers that need more development. The following is a checklist for a development strategy for carers.

Identify the carers' role:

■ within the community care plan structure;
■ in the review of service provision, for social services and health;
■ in the feedback to other departments, especially housing and finance, about the way in which their procedures affect carers.

Use assessment:

■ as a key to choice;
■ to find out whether carers are willing or able to continue caring;
■ to identify what support they need.

Develop:

■ criteria for separate assessment for carers;
■ a carers' register and consultation mechanisms;
■ your information plan;
■ areas of practical help;
■ the role of carers' groups and forums.

Establish:

■ clear, practical goals;
■ funding to support the strategy;
■ clear financial assessment and charging policies;
■ time-scales for achieving your objectives;
■ procedures for monitoring the quality of your services and the implementation of your strategy.

The importance of listening to carers

Carers want services that are reliable, flexible and certain. They are also more interested in having the opportunity for a private word with care managers than in filling in yet another form. Carers want to feel sure that messages they are giving to front-line staff are fed back to managers, so systems to allow this flow of information are very important. Carers' views and their capacity to continue caring will vary over time. You can get it right only by listening to what they are asking for.

You can play the role of an expert who knows best for your service user and find out what they need by asking questions. Alternatively, you can approach the situation as something that you both need to understand and negotiate over who might do what to help. Both approaches may end up with the carer getting what they want. The difference is in how power is used and the impact this can have on the carer. Only working together will empower the carer to be fully involved as an equal partner in a process of negotiating the nature of the problem and its possible solutions. These two approaches to dealing with people – the expert or the negotiator – are described by Smale, in *Negotiating Care in the Community*, as the Questioning model and the Exchange model.

In the *Questioning* model the professional is assumed to be the expert in identifying need. In the *Exchange* model it is assumed that everyone involved – carers, service users, professionals – has equally valid perceptions of the problems and can contribute to the solutions.

In the Questioning model you gather information, make an assessment of the needs and then determine the solution. Using the alternative Exchange model you concentrate on an exchange of information between all the parties concerned. People are, and always will be, their own expert: their situation, their relationships, what they want and need. No matter how easy or difficult it is for you to communicate with carers, they always bring their expertise about themselves and their situation to the assessment and subsequent management of the care. They will probably know what will work best when planning a care package!

KEY POINTS

- Carers see that they have common needs to which local authorities should respond.
- Carers have a legitimate concern about service provision, and can contribute to planning it effectively.

- The needs of carers from ethnic minority backgrounds are not necessarily different, but they may want them met in different ways.
- In order to involve carers fully, consultation groups need to be 'carer-friendly', bearing carers in mind when deciding when and where meetings are to be held.
- Consultation can make a difference only if you listen to carers and act on what they say.

References

Better Care, Higher Standards: A charter for long-term care, published by the Department of Health/Department of the Environment, Transport and the Regions, 1999

Carers (Recognition and Services) Act 1995 Policy Guidance, published by the Department of Health, London, 1996

Caring Today: National inspection of local authority support to carers, published by the Department of Health, London, 1995

Directory of Grant-making Trusts 1999–2000 edited by J Davis, published by Charities Aid Foundation, West Malling, Kent, 1999

Disability Rights Handbook edited by J Patterson, published by the Disability Alliance Education and Research Association, London, 1997

A Guide to Grants for Individuals in Need edited by S Harland, published by Directory of Social Change, London, 1998/9

National Strategy for Carers: Caring about carers, published by the Department of Health, London, 1999

Negotiating Care in the Community by G Smale, published by the National Institute for Social Work, London, 1992

NHS responsibilities for meeting continuing health care needs, HSG(95)5, published by the Department of Health, London, 1995

What Next for Carers? Findings from the Social Services Inspectorate project 'The Way Ahead', published by the Department of Social Services, London, 1995

4 Carers need practical help

Carers need information

Research by Carers National Association shows that carers need information.

'All I need is adequate information as to the help available.'

'Whether the information is about finances or practicalities, it's got to be somewhere accessible – the doctor's surgery would be ideal.'

'It wouldn't cost a lot to make more information available. All the members of our carers' group complain that they are not told anything – they find out by accident.'

Carers need information about:

- What caring is like in both the long and the short term.
- What help is available.
- The disease/disability of the person they are caring for.
- Nursing skills and techniques.
- Behaviour management.
- Self-help groups and associations.
- Housing.
- Money/finance/benefits.

Information needs to be given both personally and in leaflets. It must also be given in a form that can be understood. It is widely acknowledged that many people do not even realise that they *are* carers. It is important therefore to target and promote information about carers to networks where 'hidden' carers may visit; for example, community centres, pharmacies, GP surgeries, health centres, dentists, supermarkets.

Factors to consider

- Think about the language that you use. Unless someone already identifies themselves as a carer, seeing a poster or leaflet saying 'Are you a carer?' may have no meaning. Using phrases such as 'Do you look after someone?' or 'Are you worried about your mother's health?' can have more meaning for people and encourage them to come forward to find out more.
- Quality and clarity are important. Is the information correct and up to date and written in clear, jargon-free language?
- Leaflets may need to be available in languages other than English, or using other forms of communication (eg pictures such as are used for people with learning difficulties).
- Leaflets in languages other than English may be targeted to the specific communities (eg black and ethnic minority groups).
- Do not underestimate the value of word of mouth. Encourage carers you are in touch with to spread the message.
- Distribute information through community networks to as many places as possible to reach the largest number of people. Never forget the easy and the obvious: for example, the community pages in the Thomson Directory may not give any details but they offer a starting point.
- If your area has a register of carers, this can be used to distribute helpful information.
- Target and involve GPs and GP practices as far as possible.
- Target employers. Will they put a leaflet in wage packets or with salary statements?
- Target the local authority. (For example, the London Borough of Richmond includes details of carers' support and projects with the Council Tax bills.)
- Remember diversity of materials – leaflets, emergency cards, newsletters, posters.
- Send other professionals packs of information on caring and carers. This keeps the information and carers' issues at the front of

their minds; use the pack as part of the induction for new staff in social services and primary health care teams.

■ Include both general and local information in packs, as these will complement each other.

■ If you are in contact with former carers, encourage them to use their skills and experiences to support other carers.

Carers need respite

Everyone needs a break from time to time. For some people, though, the term 'respite' conjures up an image of someone needing to get away from their obligations (the *Concise Oxford Dictionary* describes the word 'respite' as *an interval of rest or relief; a delay permitted in the discharge of an obligation or the suffering of a penalty*). So carers may need support and encouragement to understand that taking a break from their daily routine of caring is not a selfish act but accepting the need for a break just the same as anyone else. It can also be helpful to encourage carers to see that taking a break will enable them to continue in their caring role. Some people find the phrase 'short term break' more neutral than 'respite care' and therefore easier to accept.

People often tend to think that 'respite' means taking a holiday for a set number of days or weeks once a year. But respite can mean a break in many different ways. It can also mean a break for the person being cared for.

This section looks at different types of respite. It invites you to think about what may be available in your area, and how carers' choice for respite can be as wide as possible. It may be offered in the following ways:

■ day and night time sitting services;
■ day centres and organised activities;
■ hospital, nursing home or hospice care;
■ residential respite care;
■ alternative care at home.

Day and night time sitting services

Sitting services provide someone who comes into the home of the person who is being cared for a few hours a week to do everything the carer would normally do, so that they can have some time off. There may be some sitting services run by the local authority, but they are often provided by voluntary organisations. One of the largest sitting schemes is the Crossroads Care Attendant Scheme (address on p 112). There are about 200 schemes across the UK, so there could be one in your area. Crossroads Care attendants are paid trained workers able to support people with high dependency needs. Other sitting services may be provided by volunteers and will not be able to be offered in all caring circumstances.

Crossroads Care services vary slightly across the UK, some providing only a day sitting service, but many more also provide a service through the night.

Knowing about the organisations that offer a sitting service in your area will be important for carers. Information about them can be found through the telephone directory, local library, local carers' projects, Council for Voluntary Service etc. The Community Service Volunteers (CSV) can often provide longer term care by matching a volunteer to 'live in' and take the place of a carer while they go away for a break.

Day centres and organised activities

There may be a number of activities available in your area for a disabled or older person. Day centres are often run by the social services department or voluntary organisations such as Age Concern. Some groups and associations run lunch clubs, drop-in centres and social activities, which can provide a welcome break for the carer as well as the person they are caring for. Local colleges also offer regular classes (eg art and crafts, languages, cookery). Residential homes for older people can provide some day care services, too.

If respite such as this can be seen as a social activity rather than 'putting a person somewhere for a few hours', it will be far more acceptable to both the carer and the person being cared for.

NHS care

If the person being cared for has complex medical needs, respite health care will be more appropriate. This will usually be provided in a hospital, nursing home or hospice but the health authority can provide or fund respite care at home. Although other forms of respite care may be charged for, no charge is made for any person who meets the health authority's criteria and is accepted as an NHS responsibility. An initial request is made to the person's GP for an assessment for respite health care. The official guidance HSG(95)5, *NHS responsibilities for meeting continuing health care needs*, sets out the details about respite health care. See also Age Concern Factsheet 37, *Hospital discharge arrangements and NHS continuing health care services*.

Hospice care

Hospices offer very specialised services, usually referred to as palliative or terminal care, when the patient's disease is not or is no longer responsive to curative treatment, and from which death is the inevitable outcome.

Hospices can offer a range of services, including outreach, day care, respite care and in-patient accommodation. Their aim is to offer the best possible quality of life to the terminally ill person, and to help them and their family and carers cope with their situation and to prepare themselves for what is ahead. The nurses and care workers involved are specially trained, and offer the support and counselling needed, in a calm and peaceful atmosphere.

Residential respite care

There will be times when the most appropriate form of respite is in a residential setting. There may not be a medical requirement, as with someone needing respite health care, but they may have a condition that leaves them confused (such as the results of a stroke or dementia), or they may have a mental illness or learning disability that makes them vulnerable. They may need attending to day and night, and there may not be a service in your area able to offer this at home.

Placing someone in residential care, even temporarily, is often a difficult step for a carer to take. The first time the person they are caring for goes into residential respite care, the carer may worry so much that they feel no benefit of the break at all. They need to be encouraged to persevere with respite care; it can help them to talk to another carer who has experienced the same feelings. Given time, they will discover that they can trust others to care for their loved ones, and that the break from each other can be of benefit to both parties.

Another consideration for the carer is the fact that they can actually have their home to themselves for a while if they wish. Having residential respite care services does not mean the carer has to go away. They could have friends to stay, instead of going to stay with them. After all, many carers cannot afford to go away but would like to be able to relax in the comfort of their home and take their time doing things such as the gardening without having to think about feeding someone else and getting them to bed.

Making use of residential respite care is also a way of gradually introducing someone to a home if they will eventually need permanent residential care.

Respite care may be offered through local authority or independent care homes. Charges will vary, depending on the level of care needed. (See also Age Concern Factsheet 10, *Local authority charging procedures for residential and nursing home care.*)

Alternative care at home

As with day and night sitting services, a number of voluntary organisations offer care at home. One already mentioned is the Crossroads Care Attendant Schemes.

Some services will provide someone to come into the home and completely replace the carer, which means doing some jobs in the home too. Others will only attend the person to be cared for, spending time talking to them, helping them with their hobbies and so on, and attending to their personal care if needed. Many carers prefer this option, particularly if the person they care for has dementia and feels more secure in familiar surroundings.

Respite is an important aspect of caring. Providing appropriate and effective respite services can mean the difference between a carer feeling able to continue in that role and remaining in reasonable health or becoming so exhausted that they either have to stop or become ill.

'If someone could have taken Mum on from time to time to help me recharge my batteries, she might not have spent the last year of her life in a home, and I might not have suffered so much stress.' A former carer of an older woman who had Alzheimer's disease

KEY POINTS

- Carers should not feel guilty because they need a break.
- A break from each other can benefit both the carer and the person they are caring for.
- 'Respite' does not mean the carer has to go away for a break.
- Respite care that incorporates leisure and hobbies helps to avoid the idea that someone is being 'put somewhere' for a few hours.

Carers may need financial help

For many people, caring has serious financial consequences. Even if a carer carries on working, they will probably find that their expenses have gone up. For example, they may have higher heating bills, additional laundry bills and special diets to cater for. If the carer has left work, they will almost certainly find it hard to make ends meet on Social Security benefits. Sometimes people are reluctant to apply for state benefits, seeing it as asking for charity. You must help them to see that the benefits are their right, not a hand-out.

You need to be well informed about any financial help a carer may be entitled to. Many carers will appreciate help with their budgeting arrangements, and this section explains how this can be done.

Benefits

The benefits system is very complicated, and most people need some help to point them in the right direction. If your knowledge of benefits is limited, carers can get information and advice from a number of other agencies, such as:

- Citizens Advice Bureaux
- Independent advice centres
- Welfare rights units
- Disablement associations
- Age Concern
- Carers National Association
- Carers' projects

Local offices or groups of the above can be found in the telephone directory, library or local authority offices.

Once a carer and the person they are caring for are receiving the financial help they are entitled to, it is important that they understand the effects of any changes in their personal situation. The changes might be in their circumstances or to the law concerning their eligibility, so carers need to ensure that they check regularly that their entitlement to help has not altered or that the kind of support provided has not changed.

Major financial problems can develop when a caring situation changes, as the following case study demonstrates.

CASE STUDY

Karen is 48 years old and single. She has been caring for her mother for 15 years, of which the last ten have been in Karen's own home.

When her mother's health deteriorated, Karen decided to give up her part-time job to enable her to care fully for her mother. She had calculated that her mother's pension and Attendance

Allowance, combined with Karen's Income Support and Invalid Care Allowance were enough to continue paying the small mortgage and cover the bills.

They managed in this way for almost six years. Then Karen's mother took a turn for the worse and her health deteriorated so much that Karen felt she could no longer give the care her mother needed. She made arrangements for her mother to move into residential care.

However, without the contribution of her mother's pension and Attendance Allowance to the household, and with the loss of the Invalid Care Allowance, Karen has found that she is unable to cover her domestic bills. After six years of unemployment, Karen has also lost confidence in her ability and doubts that she can find a job.

Attendance Allowance is a benefit intended to help with the costs of disability but can be spent in any way the recipient feels is appropriate. It is available to people over the age of 65. Before this age the equivalent benefit is included in the Disabled Living Allowance, which is divided into two components: a mobility component and a care component. The care component of the Disabled Living Allowance is equivalent to Attendance Allowance. After the age of 65 no new claims can be made to help with mobility needs (but if the Disabled Living Allowance mobility component is already being received, this will continue). In reality, most carers and the people they care for pool their resources in order to make ends meet, but they should be aware of the problems that may arise later if their circumstances change.

Benefits for carers

Carers can apply for **Invalid Care Allowance** and the **Carer Premium**.

INVALID CARE ALLOWANCE (ICA)

Invalid Care Allowance (April 1999 rate £39.95) is paid to carers under the age of 65, who care for at least 35 hours a week for someone who receives Attendance Allowance or the middle or higher rate of the Disability Living Allowance (DLA) care component. Invalid Care Allowance cannot be awarded for the first time to a carer aged 65 or over; however, if a carer qualified for this allowance before the age of 65, it will be continued when they reach 65. The carer is allowed Invalid Care Allowance if they are working, but there is an earnings limit of £50 a week at the time of writing. If the carer's earnings fluctuate, they will normally be averaged out over a period of five weeks or whatever period seems most appropriate.

For example, Jenny Smith, a nurse by profession, cares for her husband. She recently signed up with a nursing agency and does a number of night shifts for the local hospital. She earns £70 per night and, on average, works nine nights per month – three nights per week for three weeks. Although she earns nothing during the fourth week of each month, she is not entitled to Invalid Care Allowance because her earnings, when averaged out, bring her over the £50 limit.

Some expenses can be taken into account. These include child care costs and other costs of alternative care up to the value of half of the carer's net earnings in one month.

Claims for Invalid Care Allowance can be backdated only three months. So it is important that people who are new to caring are aware of their entitlement to Invalid Care Allowance and claim as soon as possible.

Warning If the person being cared for receives the Severe Disability Premium, they will lose it if the carer is awarded Invalid Care Allowance. The carer might be able to receive an extra £13.95 a week through the Carer Premium, but the person being cared for would lose a premium worth £39.75 (April 1999 rates). If the carer is unsure whether to claim Invalid Care Allowance, they should seek advice first.

Some carers may not receive Invalid Care Allowance because they are receiving another benefit such as a Widow's Pension, Incapacity Benefit or Retirement Pension (these benefits overlap with Invalid Care Allowance). It is important to note that, if the carer would be entitled to Invalid Care Allowance were it not for these other benefits and they have a low income, they may still be able to claim an additional amount as a carer – the Carer Premium.

THE CARER PREMIUM

This is not a benefit in its own right. Instead it is an extra amount (April 1999 rate £13.95) paid as part of Income Support. The premium is also included when Housing Benefit and Council Tax Benefit (Rate Rebate in Northern Ireland) are calculated.

The Carer Premium is included as part of means-tested benefits if a carer or their partner qualifies for Invalid Care Allowance – or would qualify if they were not receiving another benefit such as a Widow's Pension, Incapacity Benefit or Retirement Pension. Some carers mistakenly believe that, as they do not qualify for Invalid Care Allowance because they receive other benefits, they are not entitled to the Carer Premium either.

If both the carer and their partner qualify for Invalid Care Allowance, they can receive two Carer Premiums. Even if there is some doubt as to whether a carer is entitled to the Carer Premium, it is best to claim it anyway. If a carer applies to have the Invalid Care Allowance backdated, they may also be able to have their Carer Premium backdated.

INCOME SUPPORT

Income Support may be payable to a carer on a low income who is working fewer than 16 hours a week. Being eligible for Income Support is also a passport to other benefits, such as community care grants, Cold Weather Payments, Housing Benefit, and free NHS prescriptions, sight tests and dental treatment.

Budgeting for carers

Financial worries for carers can be very distressing and create additional stress. You are likely to come across carers who have been trying to manage for a long time and find themselves falling deeper into debt. The skill of the professional is to offer a listening ear and provide some practical support and ideas to help them sort out the problems.

There are some steps that carers can take to help maximise their income and minimise their outgoings. The following information is available to carers in 'Money Worries', an information sheet from Carers National Association.

HELPING TO MAXIMISE INCOME

- Check that the carer and the person they are caring for are receiving their full benefit entitlements.
- The carer and their partner should check their Income Tax position. People on a low income do not have to pay tax and can apply to receive interest payments on savings paid in full. (Normally tax is deducted automatically at source.) They should also check whether they are receiving their full tax allowances. Free advice about tax is available at local tax offices or advice centres.
- If the person being cared for has been in an accident, it may be worth seeking legal advice to see if they can get compensation through the courts. People on a low income may get help through Legal Aid to pay the legal costs.
- Most benefits allow people to do some part-time work without affecting their eligibility. Some carers may be able to consider part-time work, working from home or renting out a spare room, but make sure they get advice first.
- Think about other people who are living in the same house, such as adult children. Are they contributing enough to the household?
- If a carer has a bill they cannot meet, there may be a charity that can help out. There is a book available at most libraries, called *A Guide to Grants for Individuals in Need*.

HELPING TO MINIMISE OUTGOINGS

- The cost of fuel and other bills can be spread over the year through budget schemes or by buying savings stamps at the post office. This can help avoid getting large bills in the winter.
- The carer should make sure they are not spending money on things they could get help with: prescription charges, free school meals etc.
- Good insulation in the home can help reduce heating bills. Sometimes grants for home insulation are available to people on low incomes or who are receiving Income Support or Working Families Credit. The Home Energy Efficiency Scheme grant is available to anyone over 60 and receiving an income-related benefit, towards the installation of energy-conservation measures. (For more information, contact the Energy Action Grants Agency Ltd – address on p 113.)

DEALING WITH DEBTS

Carers may have to repay debts such as rent arrears and credit charges. They may need reassurance that even the worst muddle can usually be sorted out with advice from a money adviser. The Citizens Advice Bureau can put people in touch with money advisers. Many companies are prepared to accept very small weekly payments while the carer is in difficulties, and will sometimes waive interest charges.

Renovation and disabled facilities grants

A carer may be able to get some help with the cost of improving, repairing or adapting their home. This makes financial sense and ensures that the carer and the person they are caring for are able to live in a safe and secure environment.

Grants are available from the local authority housing or environmental health departments. They can be either *mandatory*, meaning that the local authority is obliged to provide the grant, or *discretionary*, which means that grants can be awarded if the local authority feels it is reasonable to do so.

Discretionary renovation grants (for repair work) are available under the Housing Grants, Construction and Regeneration Act 1996. They are usually granted only to tenants and owners who have been in residence for at least three years before they make an application.

Disabled facilities grants are mandatory. They are designed to help make the home of a disabled person more suitable, and to help the person manage more independently. Carers who are living with a disabled person can apply. Works covered by this grant include:

- Improving access to get in and out of the home.
- Improving access to the bedroom, kitchen, bathroom, living room.
- Providing suitable bathroom and kitchen facilities.
- Adapting heating or lighting controls.

To receive the grant, a means test is carried out on the disabled person and their husband or wife, but **not** the carer if it is someone different but living in the same home (eg the carer of an older parent). Unfortunately, payment of this grant can sometimes be delayed for up to 12 months.

Home Repair Assistance is a scheme designed to help older or disabled people carry out small repairs. This grant is discretionary.

Note No work should be carried out until the grant has been approved. Anything done before approval will not be covered.

Council Tax

Council Tax is a tax on property, determined by the local authority's valuation of the home, but the size of the bill also depends on how many people over the age of 18 are living there.

The principle behind the Council Tax system is that the average household consists of two people and that a two-person household with an average income will pay a full bill. There are discounts if there is only one person in the household. People living alone pay 25 per cent less than a full bill. If no one at all lives in the property, the bill is reduced by 50 per cent.

Some properties are completely exempt from Council Tax. For example, if a carer lives alone in a flat but goes to stay with their mother to look after her, the flat is exempt. If the mother leaves her home to be cared for by the carer in the carer's flat, her property is exempt.

When counting how many people live in a house, certain people are ignored completely. They are 'invisible' in the count. Carers are included in this group but only if they are living with and caring for a disabled person who is not their husband, wife, cohabitee (partner) or child under 18. The disabled person must receive the higher rate of Attendance Allowance or the Disability Living Allowance care component, and the carer must be providing at least 35 hours of care a week. So a person caring for their father could qualify, but a person caring for their spouse or 17-year-old child would not.

Other 'invisible' people include:

- People in prison and people detained under the Mental Health Act.
- People who are severely mentally impaired (eg people with dementia).
- Children and people over the age of 18 who are still at school.
- Full-time students, apprentices, trainees and student nurses.
- People who live in hospital, a nursing home or residential care.
- Live-in care workers provided by a charity (eg Community Service Volunteers).

If a carer living with his or her mother qualifies as an 'invisible' person, the mother would be seen as a single occupant and the property would get a 25 per cent discount. However, if the mother had dementia, she too would be considered 'invisible', and the property would get a 50 per cent reduction.

Remember that there are also reductions and rebates available to people on a low income. For example, Fred and John are joint tenants. The joint Council Tax bill is £200. If Fred is on Income Support, the local authority will set a rebate of £100; if John has a low income, he can apply for a rebate on the basis of his £100 share of the bill (*source*: Carers National Association Information sheet).

The designated banding of the property can also be affected if there are adaptations or additional facilities for a disabled person. Where this is the case, the band charge is lowered by one level; for Band A properties the charge is reduced by one-sixth.

KEY POINTS

- The benefits system is very complicated. Unless you have regular training on all benefits, refer carers to an expert for benefits advice.
- Make sure that carers are aware of the implications of 'pooling resources' in order to support the household.
- Many carers would welcome practical support and advice on maximising their income and minimising outgoings.
- Many carers are reluctant to claim for benefits. Reassure them that this is not charity but what they are rightfully entitled to.
- If there is any doubt about whether someone is eligible for a benefit, they should claim it. They will be told if they are not eligible. However, if a carer has not been claiming a benefit but could have done so a long time ago, they may lose out because most cannot be backdated very far.

Help with transport and getting about

Carers often find themselves isolated because they do not have the transport facilities appropriate to them or the person they are caring for. There are a number of facilities designed to enable people travel more easily. Schemes vary across the UK, but the following information (listed in alphabetical order) may help you to find out what is available in your area. See also Age Concern Factsheet 26: *Travel information for older people*.

Hospital transport Ambulances or cars are used for hospital appointments by people who are medically unfit to travel any other way, and must be authorised by a doctor. However, other services are available, which may be charged for. Ask the GP, hospital or local volunteer bureau for details of any services in your area.

Buses Many local authorities (the district council or the borough council in London, other cities and urban areas) operate a concessionary fares scheme for older and disabled people. Reduced fares are usually available Monday to Friday after 9am and all day at the weekend and on Bank Holidays. In some areas, buses with a lower or more easily accessible door now operate. Contact local bus operators for details.

Disability Living Allowance: mobility component This is a non-means-tested, tax-free allowance for people aged 5 to 65 with mobility problems. (A claim must be made before the person's 65th birthday is reached. If someone is in receipt of this benefit before the age of 65, their entitlement continues after their 65th birthday.) The local Benefits Agency can provide details and claim forms.

Disabled Person's Railcard This railcard offers reduced fares for certain categories of passengers, giving up to one-third off a range of rail tickets. An application form and a booklet called *Rail Travel for Disabled Passengers* can be obtained from most staffed stations or from the address on page 113.

Mobility Advice and Vehicle Information Service (MAVIS) This organisation (address on p 114) provides practical advice on driving, car adaptations and car choice for disabled drivers and passengers.

Motability This voluntary organisation (address on p 115) helps individuals to purchase a car with adaptations, using the mobility component of the Disability Living Allowance.

Orange Badge Scheme Now called the Blue Badge Scheme, this allows disabled people to park closer to the shops or other restricted areas, whether they are the driver or the passenger. Application forms are available from the local social services department.

Post bus services These involve the postman/woman picking up passengers on their delivery round. The service is sometimes available in villages with no other public transport. Information on what is available can usually be found in the local library, or through the Royal Mail Postbus unit.

Sea and air travel It is best to inform the airline or shipping company direct, in advance, of any special needs there may be. This can be done through a travel agent but it is advisable to confirm arrangements with the company direct.

Taxi companies All district councils have a legal obligation to register a taxi company with vehicles able to take wheelchairs. Contact your local authority for details.

Trains Help is available with wheelchairs, space on trains, transfer between platforms and, in London, transfer between mainline stations. It is best to try to plan the journey in advance with the nearest staffed train station.

Tripscope This voluntary organisation (address on p 118) can supply travel and transport information for older and disabled people in London and the southwest of England.

Vehicle Excise Duty Exemption (road tax) Some people who receive the higher mobility component of the Disability Living Allowance can claim exemption from road tax. Applicants should write to the Mobility Allowance Unit (address on p 115).

Volunteer bureaux These may provide a transport scheme, in which mileage is charged. Find out from the National Association of Volunteer Bureaux (address on p 116) what is available in your area.

Carers' support groups

Carers need the opportunity to meet other carers. The unique support that they receive from each other gives a particular and special nature to carers' groups. Research by Carers National Association in 1986, into the effectiveness of carers' support groups, revealed that carers gain more from them than they at first expect. It also showed that groups are seen as a lifeline by many carers. Moreover, they often find that they are given the confidence to speak up for themselves and other carers. Their involvement in carers' forums, consultation conferences, planning groups and so on has ensured that carers' issues and insights have remained high on local social and political agendas.

Carers' support groups can offer:

- The chance to meet people in similar circumstances.
- A break, however short, from caring responsibilities.
- Information.
- Support.

There are two main types of carers' groups. There are specialist groups for carers of people with a particular condition. They are often affiliated to one of the national voluntary organisations representing people in a similar situation, such as MENCAP or the Alzheimer's Society. These can offer a great deal of information and specific training both for the carer and for the person being cared for.

The other type is a general support group for all carers, in which the emphasis is much more on the needs of the carers themselves. Carers may just meet for a chat and a cup of tea, or they might invite someone to come to talk to them about something totally unrelated to caring. Or occasionally they might arrange to go shopping together or out for a meal. Groups vary according to the needs of the members, but usually the emphasis is on mutual support, sharing experiences and information, relaxing in the company of people who understand their situation, and even having a little fun.

Setting up a carers' group

Having made contact with a few carers, you may feel that it is feasible to set up a carers' support group. Before you start, try to obtain support from other bodies. For example, talk to Carers National Association (address on p 111) and see if there are any other local projects that could help or advise.

A date, time and place for the first meeting need to be decided. This meeting may be in someone's home – it is often more informal and people find it easier to relax. At the first meeting the group members will have to agree:

- How often to meet (many groups meet monthly, some more often, some less).

- Whether to vary between daytime and evening meetings to allow more people to come.
- Where to meet: small groups may find it most convenient to meet in someone's home but larger groups often find that their local social services department or health centre will let them use a room for meetings free of charge.
- How to keep in touch between meetings.
- Confidentiality. It is important to treat what members say with respect and not to discuss other people's personal experiences without their permission. Members will not feel happy to talk if they fear that what they say may be discussed outside the group. It is important to agree this at the outset and make it clear to new members.

Other factors that will need to be considered:

Meeting arrangements	Arranging a timetable Finding a venue Booking the room Refreshments Contacting the speaker
Transport	If carers have difficulty in travelling to meetings, you may need a lift rota; or there might be a community transport service that could be used
Respite care	Members may need a sitter to enable them to go to meetings – there may be a local scheme such as Crossroads, or the local social services department may run a service
Newsletter	Carers who find it difficult to attend meetings regularly can appreciate receiving a newsletter to keep in touch with the group activities
Fundraising	Most groups need little money to run them, particularly if free accommodation for the meetings can be arranged and the cost of refreshments is shared. However, if a newsletter is produced, money will be needed for photocopying and postage

'It really helped to be able to talk to someone who understood what caring is like.' A 'new' carer after attending his first carers' support group meeting

KEY POINTS

- Research has shown that carers gain more from support groups than they first expected.
- Support groups can help a carer to realise that they are not alone.
- Groups will vary according to the needs of their members, but usually the emphasis is on mutual support.

References and further reading

Age Concern Factsheets:

10: *Local authority charging procedures for residential and nursing home care*

13: *Older home owners: financial help with repairs and adaptations*

16: *Income related benefits: income and capital*

17: *Housing Benefit and Council Tax Benefit*

18: *A brief guide to money benefits*

21: *The Council Tax and older people*

25: *Income Support and the Social Fund*

26: *Travel information for older people*

34: *Attendance Allowance and Disability Living Allowance*

37: *Hospital discharge arrangements and NHS continuing health care services*

A Guide to Grants for Individuals in Need edited by S Harland, published by Directory of Social Change, London, 1998/9

NHS responsibilities for meeting continuing health care needs HSG(95)5, published by the Department of Health, London, 1995

Speak Up, Speak Out: Research amongst members of Carers National Association, published by Carers National Association, London, 1992

5 Specific needs of ethnic groups

Understanding the issues

Many different races, cultures and religions make up British society today. This diversity enriches and enhances the social fabric of the nation. It is also a diversity that defies glib and all-embracing generalisations.

Some ethnic minority communities comprise people with origins in one area of a country and are very close-knit. Other people from within the ethnic minority populations do not belong to a 'community' at all. Both within and among communities there are often differing approaches to medicine and healing, differing views of illness, disability and old age, and differing responses to the responsibilities and tasks of caring.

People providing services should be cautious about making assumptions about the needs of ethnic minority people. A common assumption among many service providers is that there is an extended family, particularly for Asian and Chinese families, which will prefer to take the responsibility for long-term care and is in a position to do this. This may be true for some, but it is far from the case for many people. The immigration process itself affects the make-up of the extended family. In addition, many aspects of life in modern Britain weaken family networks or their capacity to provide sufficient support and care. This is borne out by a recent report from the Social Services Inspectorate: *They Look After Their Own, Don't They?*

Racism

It should not be assumed that, because people do not come forward for services such as day care or home help, these are neither needed nor wanted. The content of services and the ways in which they are provided may not reflect the variety of people's needs and the realities of their lives. Above all, these realities include discrimination and racism.

- There is the racism of a 'colour-blind' approach to service delivery, where people from ethnic minorities are expected to fit into existing services although their needs may require specific responses. For example, not telling people in their mother tongue about respite services that are available excludes many who do not have English as their first language.
- There is also the more obvious racism that continues to see people as immigrants in Britain, thus considering their stay in this country as temporary. This damaging view does not accept, for example, British-born black people as permanently resident here and therefore entitled to services. The 1991 Census figures show that at least 50 per cent of the black population today were born in Britain.

Providing support

The needs of people from ethnic minorities are no different from those of everyone else in society. They, too, need information, respite care, practical help, someone to talk to, financial support and so forth, as explored in the other chapters of this book. The issues that arise are to do with obtaining equal access to these services and equal treatment. *Caring for Ethnic Minority Elders* by Yasmin Alibhai-Brown gives the background of the main ethnic minority communities in the UK, and outlines some of the possible variations in culture that we should be aware of. *Culture, Religion and Patient Care in a Multiethnic Society* by Alix Henley and Judith Schott gives more detailed information with particular reference to health care.

Providing a service that is responsive to the diverse needs of different sections of the community is likely to require developments in the following areas.

Sensitivity and responsiveness

Professionals need to give attention to each family's circumstances when planning the services to be provided. For some families it will be important to ensure that staff are themselves from the relevant minority community, or at least of the same gender. Greater consultation may be needed as well as continual monitoring and review to ensure that services are and remain appropriate.

Specific services

People from minority groups may feel more comfortable with services that are focused not only on the condition but also on people from a similar background. The response to supporting people from ethnic minorities is often to provide 'special' services that are seen as appropriate and helpful. Calling these services 'special' may contribute to the view that people from ethnic minorities are a problematic group requiring additional resources from an already over-stretched budget. Perhaps it helps to consider support requested as 'specific' rather than 'special'. For instance, offering a sitting service where staff members speak Punjabi or providing a prayer room for Muslim users in a day centre is by no means special, but certainly a specific response.

When working with carers of a cultural background different from your own, it is important to be aware of potential barriers to communication and understanding. If your area of work includes ethnic minority communities, you should ensure that you have relevant information about their culture, religious beliefs, family expectations and history. Local community centres, services and places of worship can often be very helpful in developing your knowledge and understanding. Remember, though, not to assume that everyone from a particular ethnic community will necessarily follow all – or indeed any – of that society's beliefs. Everyone, whatever their background, is an individual and should be treated as such.

If the carer's first language is not English, this may pose some difficulties. You must consider carefully how to make sure that all parties understand what is going on. This can present quite a challenge, as the following case study shows.

CASE STUDY

Mrs Singh cares for her husband who was recently involved in an industrial accident, leaving him physically disabled and in need of a high level of personal care. They have four young children. Mrs Singh's parents also live with the family. The care manager, Clare Rudd, had already been involved in an assessment for Mr Singh jointly with the medical team before his discharge from hospital two weeks earlier, and certain items of equipment are being installed to enable him to have some mobility in the home. Even though Mr and Mrs Singh speak little English, that assessment had been relatively straightforward, largely due to the assistance of Mr Singh's consultant, who provided the interpretation needed to communicate.

At the time of her husband's assessment, Mrs Singh asked if she could have a carer's assessment at a later stage when everyone had settled into some sort of routine. Clare arranged to visit the family in their home at a later date. This would also give her the opportunity to see how things were going for them.

Clare has been concerned that there would be a language barrier without the help of the consultant, but she understands that Mr and Mrs Singh's ten-year-old son Tilak can speak fluent English and will be able to interpret for them.

On her arrival at Mr and Mrs Singh's home, Clare discovers that Mrs Singh does not want her son to be the interpreter, but is reluctant to explain why in his presence. Eventually, Clare leaves without giving the carer's assessment but makes an appointment to return in two weeks.

It turned out that Mrs Singh wanted to discuss something of a personal nature about the care of Mr Singh. It would have been very inappropriate for a young boy to have been involved in such a discussion, particularly as it concerned his father.

Clare then discovered that Mr Singh's sister, who lives in the next town, can speak and understand English.

> Clare returns two weeks later ready to discuss the carer's assessment with Mrs Singh, via her sister-in-law Hardev. However, it soon becomes clear to Clare that at times Hardev expresses her own opinion of the caring situation rather than her sister's. In order to conduct a full and fair assessment for Mrs Singh, Clare finds an independent advocate through a translation service.

Clare would have avoided these frustrations had she been aware of the problems that can be caused by language and cultural barriers.

As well as being aware of the barriers to communication, the care professional should also be careful not to make assumptions about family expectations – mainly that the extended family (aunts, uncles, grandparents, etc) all live under one roof and provide support for each other. Remember the following points:

- Many people live in smaller houses unable to accommodate large families.
- More women now have jobs, full- or part-time, outside the home.
- Although their ethnic origin may be Asian, Caribbean, African or elsewhere, two or three generations are now British-born, and have adopted a mixed culture.

In order to preserve people's cultural heritage, services should be designed to be able to to meet the needs of carers of ethnic minority backgrounds and those they care for.

Information

Access to information is a problem for everyone, but people from ethnic minorities often live in greater isolation than others, especially when they speak little English. The following are some suggestions about ways that may help to overcome this.

Providing translation

Translations must be available in appropriate languages and in an understandable form. Information on how to get services and how to complain should be given particular attention. Complex legal language about benefits and procedures, or difficult medical terminology, often do not translate well. Translations should be developed in consultation with relevant minority groups. The existence of such information needs to be well publicised.

Newsletters

Newsletters in relevant languages can be useful in disseminating information to ethnic minority carers.

Alternatives to the written word

Alternatives to the written word need to be explored. Some ethnic minority carers have received only a limited education or may be unable to read and write in their own language. The use of ethnic minority community radio in some cities can offer direct contact with housebound carers whose understanding of English is limited. Audio-cassette tapes, which can be played in carers' own homes, are another way of producing information. These should be well publicised.

Video films

Video films targeted at specific groups can explain a range of services to carers; for example, chiropody or continence services. Some social services departments have made progress in this area and there are several informative videos aimed at the needs of minority communities. Scope (a project for Asian elders in Leicester) and Leicester Council for Voluntary Service have jointly developed a video for carers. Videos should be well publicised and made available for viewing in community centres, day centres and residential homes.

Home visits

Home visits bringing information may be needed by some carers. These could be done by people who are working with carers or by someone who speaks their language and is likely to have some understanding of their circumstances.

Use of schools

Another route for some families is through written materials given to children to bring home from school. This may give it added importance and, even when in English, can be read either by someone else in the family or by a neighbour or friend.

Presentation of information

Posters and other illustrative material should include all races and backgrounds; for example, using photographs of Asian, Afro-Caribbean and Chinese people. In addition, publicity materials might explicitly encourage ethnic minority carers, and the people they care for, to take up services.

KEY POINTS

- Although all people's basic needs are similar, professionals should learn about cultural or religious differences that could affect the way services are delivered to someone from an ethnic minority.
- Carers from ethnic minority communities may need specific consideration to prevent difficulties in communication.
- Remember that everyone is an individual, regardless of their ethnic background.

References

Caring for Ethnic Minority Elders by Yasmin Alibhai-Brown, published by Age Concern England, London, 1998

Culture, Religion and Patient Care in a Multi-ethnic Society by Alix Henley and Judith Schott, published by Age Concern England, London, 1999

They Look After Their Own, Don't They? Inspection of community care services for black and ethnic minority older people, published by the Social Services Inspectorate, London, 1998

EPILOGUE

Carers are the mainstay of community care, and the crucial element in the care of your service users or patients. We hope that this handbook will help you to maintain and improve the relationship between the unpaid and the paid professionals – the carer and the care worker, care manager, GP and staff, and so on.

The support of carers is a vast topic that is subject to constant change. Indeed, by the time you read this book, some changes will have taken place in terms of views, attitudes and information. And there will always be people who are new to caring.

We hope that you will be able to make use of the ideas, suggestions and information given here, and that the book will help you to develop your own creative and successful methods of supporting your partners in care – family carers.

APPENDIX 1

Local authority charging procedures for residential and nursing home care

The information that follows has been extracted from Age Concern factsheets. It describes the financial help that may be available from the local authority for older people needing residential or nursing home care. For more details, see Age Concern Factsheet 10: *Local authority charging procedures for residential and nursing home care.*

This appendix is correct at the time of going to press. However, it is not a complete guide to the law, which is, in any event, subject to change from time to time. It is important, therefore, that you always make sure that you are up to date with the latest developments, which may affect the information you pass on to carers.

Who pays for the costs of a place in a care home?

Most people will be expected to pay from their own income and capital towards the costs of their care in residential or nursing homes. But some people may have their care paid for by the NHS through their local health authority.

Since 1 April 1996, each health authority must publish its own criteria for providing a range of services for people with continuing physical or mental health care needs. These services include NHS continuing in-patient care, which the health authority can provide either in an NHS hospital or nursing home or by paying for a place in a private nursing home. The health authority will use its criteria to decide whether a person is eligible for any continuing health care services from the NHS – which is 'free at the point of use'.

If someone's need for continuing health care is arranged and paid for in full by their health authority, they will be considered to be an NHS patient. In such an instance, benefits such as state retirement pension, Income Support or Attendance Allowance will reduce or stop in time. But the individual will not have to pay for NHS care from other income such as an occupational or personal pension or from capital.

How do people qualify for state financial help?

The information below is about the way means-testing will be applied if a place in a care home is not being paid for by the NHS.

Whether someone's stay in a care home is temporary or permanent, getting financial support from the local authority will depend first on the social services department assessing that person and then deciding that they need a place in a residential or nursing home.

The means test

The means test is a charging procedure, and is also called a *financial assessment*. It is the system for calculating how much a person should contribute towards the costs of their care in a home. This always applies if they enter a home permanently, and it may apply if they are resident only temporarily (eg for respite care). If a person cannot pay the standard rate – the amount it costs the local authority to provide the place – a means test must be carried out. Some local authorities make use of a rule that allows them to charge a 'reasonable amount' for up to eight weeks rather than carry out the means test. After eight weeks, though, they must assess the resident's ability to pay.

Anyone who has capital above £16,000 will be deemed to be able to pay the 'standard rate'. People whose capital is between £10,000 and £16,000 will be expected to make some contribution from their capital as well as from their income. Capital below £10,000 is ignored and not included in the means test, but a person with this amount will still be expected to contribute from their income.

The rules that local authorities have to follow are closely linked to, but not exactly the same as, the means test for Income Support.

Permanent residents

CAPITAL

Most forms of capital and savings will be counted in the means test, including bank or building society accounts, National Savings accounts, Premium Bonds, stocks and shares, and property. The surrender value of a life insurance policy, though, will be ignored.

If a resident has more than £16,000 in capital, they will be expected to pay the full fee until the amount of the capital falls to £16,000 or less. However, no one whose place is arranged by the local authority is expected to pay more than the standard rate, whatever their income or capital.

If the capital is between £10,000 and £16,000, this will be assessed as showing an assumed (or 'tariff') income. Every £250, or part of £250, of capital between £10,000 and £16,000 will be assessed as though there were an extra £1 a week income. For example, capital of £12,300 will be treated as extra income of £10 a week. Contributions should be reviewed each time the capital moves into another £250 'band'.

If someone's capital is less than £10,000, it is assumed that there is no income from this.

As with income, only capital in the name of the person going into the care home should be included in the means test. If capital is held jointly with someone else, only half of this amount will be assessed. This also includes bank and building society accounts held jointly: only half of the balance in the account will be included as capital to be assessed. In such circumstances, it may be well to advise a service user to consider splitting joint accounts into two equal separate accounts. This is because it is always half of the *balance* of the account that is counted; it is not possible, for the purpose of the means test, to 'spend down' only one-half of a joint account.

THE VALUE OF A PERSON'S HOME

The value of a person's home will be treated as capital, less 10 per cent of that value if expenses would be incurred in selling it.

Nevertheless, there are instances when the value of the person's home must be ignored for the purpose of the means test. They are ignored when it continues to be lived in by one or more of the following:

- a spouse or partner;
- a relative who is aged 60 or over;
- a relative who is under 60 but is disabled;
- a child under the age of 16 who is maintained by the person entering the care home.

The local authority has discretion to ignore the value of the home if it will continue to be lived in by someone who does not fit into the categories listed above – for example, a younger relative who is not disabled but has been the carer.

Jointly owned property can be complicated. The local authority must assess the resident's interest in it, which will depend on whether anyone would be willing to buy the resident's share. Guidance about this is given in the Department of Health's _Charging for residential accommodation guide_ (CRAG), paragraphs 7.012–7.014.

The means test calculations

Once the local authority has all the relevant information on income and savings, it can calculate how much should be contributed by a service user towards the cost of their care. In calculating what someone should pay, the local authority should make sure that the person has a _personal expenses allowance_ (or PEA). At the time of writing this allowance is £14.75 per week. The user should always receive, in writing, an explanation of how the costs have been calculated.

References

Age Concern Factsheet 10: _Local authority charging procedures for residential and nursing home care_

Charging for residential accommodation guide (CRAG), paragraphs 7.012–7.014, published by the Department of Health, London

APPENDIX 2

Challenging a decision

This appendix explains what a person can do if they do not agree with the results of their assessment or do not like the service(s) they have been offered. The information has been taken from Age Concern Factsheet 32: *Disability and ageing: your rights to social services.*

Local authority complaints procedure

People have a right to complain to the local authority, which must have a formal complaints procedure that is explained to them (Local Authority Services Act 1970, section 7B, as defined in section 50 of the National Health Service and Community Care Act 1990). This can include complaining when the local authority has assessed a person as not needing a service but the person believes that they do need it, as well as complaining about the service(s) offered.

The circumstances in which a carer has a right to complain in respect of their own carer's assessment (under the Carers Act 1995) depend on the assessment of the person they are caring for. If the person they are caring for is *not* about to have an assessment or a re-assessment, the carer has no right to an assessment of their own. However, when the person being cared for is having an assessment, the local authority has a *duty* to provide one for the carer, if requested.

Each local authority will have its own complaints procedure, and you should be familiar with it.

The local government ombudsman

If no satisfaction has been obtained through the complaints procedure, the local government ombudsman can be approached if a service user or carer feels that there has been maladministration by the local authority. 'Maladministration' covers faults in the way something has been done. It can include neglect, unjustified delay, unfair discrimination or failure to abide by agreed procedures or to have proper procedures.

The complaint can be made direct to the ombudsman or through a councillor. It must be made within 12 months after the local authority's decision. If the ombudsman decides to investigate, the investigation may take a long time. Any recommendations from the ombudsman are not binding, and the local authority can choose to ignore them. However, the ombudsman's report is made public. The address of the relevant ombudsman can be obtained from the local authority, a library or the Citizens Advice Bureau.

Appeal to the Secretary of State for Health

If a person thinks that the local authority has a duty to provide them with a service it will not provide, or that it unfairly withdrew that service, they – or someone acting on their behalf – can report the local authority to the Secretary of State for Health (Local Authority Social Services Act 1970 as amended by section 50 of the National Health Service and Community Care Act 1990). They should not do this until after going through the local authority's own complaints procedure, and they may wish to consult a solicitor for advice and to be sure that they have a case before wasting time and effort.

Appeal through the courts

Another route is to proceed through the courts but a solicitor would need to be consulted. It is possible for people to get Legal Aid if they are on a low income.

A local authority can be sued for a *breach of its statutory duty*, which can be difficult to prove. It involves a person showing:

■ a specific need for which they think services should be provided;
■ which service or services is/are required to satisfy the need;
■ that they have asked for the service(s); and
■ that the local authority has failed to satisfy the need.

A *judicial review* of the local authority's action can be requested in the High Court. In this case, the court can be asked to examine whether the local authority's action has been legal, rational and reasonable. The main grounds for challenging the local authority's action are:

- *Illegality* – the authority got the law wrong.
- *Irrationality* – the authority acted unreasonably in making its decision.
- *Procedural impropriety* – the authority did not follow correct procedures and/or did not take into account all relevant considerations, including representations from the person affected.

The procedure for a judicial review is in two stages: application is made for 'leave to apply' for judicial review; if this is granted, the case will be heard. There is evidence that some local authorities have reversed decisions on threat of legal action, particularly after leave to apply has been granted.

Reference

Age Concern Factsheet 32: *Disability and ageing: your rights to social services*

USEFUL ADDRESSES

Age Concern
See page 120

Alzheimer's Society
Gordon House
10 Greencoat Place
London SW1P 1PH
Tel: 020 7306 0606

Advice and information to carers and families of people with dementia. There are over 300 groups and contacts in England, Wales and Northern Ireland.

Alzheimer's Scotland – Action on Dementia
8 Hill Street
Edinburgh EH2 3JZ
Tel: 0131 220 4886

Advice and information in Scotland to carers and families of people with dementia.

Anchor Trust
Fountain Court
Oxford Spires Business Park
Kidlington
Oxon OX5 1NX
Tel: 01865 854000

Housing and care for older people in England. There are sheltered housing, residential care and services to help older home owners to improve and adapt their homes.

Arthritis Care
18 Stephenson Way
London NW1 2HD
Tel: 020 7916 1500
Freephone helpline: 0808 800 4050 (Monday–Friday 12–4pm)

Information, counselling, training, fun and social contact. The first port of call for anyone with arthritis. There are many smaller organisations for particular types of arthritis. Arthritis Care's helpline can provide details.

Association of Charity Officers
Beechwood House
Wyllyotts Close
Potters Bar
Hertfordshire EN6 2HW
Tel: 01707 651777

Information about charities that make grants to individuals in need.

Association for Spina Bifida and Hydrocephalus (ASBAH)
42 Park Road
Peterborough PE1 2UQ
Tel: 01733 555988
Fax: 01733 555985

Practical help and information to people with spina bifida and/or hydrocephalus, and their families. Trained fieldworkers visit families, and specialist advisers help with mobility, continence, education, etc. There is also the **Scottish Spina Bifida Association**.

Benefits Agency
See your local telephone directory
Responsible for paying Social Security benefits; provides advice through local offices.

British Association for Counselling
1 Regent Place
Rugby
Warwickshire CV21 2PJ
Tel: 01788 550899

To find out about counselling services in your area.

British Epilepsy Association
40 Hanover Square
Leeds LS3 1BE
Tel: 0113 243 9393
Fax: 0113 242 8804

Regional groups and branches, and a regional office in Belfast. The Association provides community care for people with epilepsy. (See also Epilepsy Association of Scotland.)

Care and Repair Ltd
Castle House
Kirtley Drive
Nottingham NG7 1LD
Tel: 0115 979 9091

Advice on home improvements and grants. Co-ordinates about 150 home improvement agencies country-wide that help older or disabled people, who may be living on a low income, to repair or adapt their homes.

Carers National Association
20–25 Glasshouse Yard
London EC1A 4JS
Tel: 020 7490 8818
Carers Helpline 0345 573369 (a low-cost call) (Monday–Friday 10am–noon, 2–4pm)

Advice and support for carers. It campaigns for services, enables carers to speak out and provides a network of carers' support groups.

Charity Search
25 Portview Road
Avonmouth
Bristol BS11 9LD
Tel: 0118 982 4060

Information about possible sources of financial help for older people.

Chartered Society of Physiotherapy
14 Bedford Row
London WC1R 4ED
Tel: 020 7242 1941

For chartered physiotherapists in your area.

Community Service Volunteers
237 Pentonville Road
London N1 9NJ
Tel: 020 7278 6601

Creates opportunities for volunteer work.

Contact the Elderly
15 Henrietta Street
London WC2E 8QH
Tel: 020 7240 0630

Provides companions for housebound people.

Crossroads Care Attendant Schemes
10 Regent Place
Rugby
Warwickshire CV21 2PN
Tel: 01788 573653

Volunteers to help care for someone at home.

CRUSE – Bereavement Care
126 Sheen Road
Richmond
Surrey TW9 1UR
Tel: 020 8940 4818

Bereavement advice and support. Local branches give practical advice and provide individual and group counselling and opportunities for social contact.

Department of Health
PO Box 410
Wetherby LS23 7LN
Tel: 01937 840250

For their publications (eg policy guidance and practice guides).

DIAL UK (Disablement Information and Advice Lines)
Park Lodge
St Catherine's Hospital
Tickhill Road
Balby
Doncaster DN4 8QN
Tel: 01302 310123

Information and advice for people with disabilities. Has a network of disability advice centres in England, run by people with direct experience of disability.

Disability Alliance
1st Floor East
Universal House
88–94 Wentworth Street
London E1 7SA
Tel: 020 7247 8776

Information about welfare benefits.

Disabled Person's Railcard Office
PO Box 1YT
Newcastle-upon-Tyne NE99 1YT
Helpline: 0191 269 0303

For a railcard offering concessionary fares. Application form and booklet *Rail Travel for Disabled Passengers* can be found at most staffed stations or from the address above.

Down's Syndrome Association
153–155 Mitcham Road
London SW17 9PG
Tel: 020 8682 4001

Support for people with Down's syndrome and their families, with branches and groups throughout England, Wales and Northern Ireland. (See also **Scottish Down's Syndrome Association**.)

Energy Action Grants Agency Ltd
Freepost
PO Box 130
Newcastle-upon-Tyne NE99 2RP
Tel: 0800 181 667 or 0800 072 0150
Textphone: 0800 072 1056

Administers the Home Energy Efficiency Scheme.

Epilepsy Association of Scotland
48 Govan Road
Glasgow G51 1JL
Tel: 0141 427 4911
Fax: 0141 427 7414

Supports a network of branches, groups and professional staff at resource centres in Scotland.

Headway (National Head Injuries Association)
7 King Edward Court
King Edward Street
Nottingham NG1 1EW
Tel: 0115 924 0800

Advice and information to people with a head injury; some day care services. There are 108 local groups throughout the country.

Holiday Care Service
2 Old Bank Chambers
Station Road
Horley
Surrey RH6 9HW
Tel: 01293 774535

Information and advice about holidays for older or disabled people, one-parent families and those disadvantaged by low income.

Law Centres Federation
18 Warren Street
London W1P 5DB
Tel: 020 7387 8570
Fax: 020 7387 8368

Promotes the 55 law centres located throughout the UK, which provide independent, free legal advice and representation to people living in the area.

MAVIS (Mobility Advice and Vehicle Information Service)
Transport Road Research Laboratory
Old Wokingham Road
Crowthorne
Berkshire RG45 6AU
Tel: 01344 661000

Advice on car adaptations and transport for disabled people.

MENCAP (Royal Society for Mentally Handicapped Children and Adults)
National Centre
123 Golden Lane
London EC1Y 0RT
Tel: 020 7454 0454

Advice and support for people with a learning disability and their families and carers.

MIND (National Association for Mental Health)
Granta House
15–19 Broadway
London E15 4BQ
Tel: 020 8519 2122

Advice and support for people with mental health problems and their families and friends. Services range from counselling to housing projects. There are over 230 local associations throughout Britain.

Mobility Allowance Unit
North Fylde
Central Office
Norcross
Blackpool FY5 3TA
Tel: 0345 123456 (a low-cost call)

For people receiving the higher mobility component of the Disability Living Allowance to claim exemption from car road tax.

Motability
2nd floor
Gate House
Westgate
Harlow
Essex CM20 1HR
Tel: 01279 635660

Helps individuals purchase a car with adaptations, using the mobility component of their Disability Living Allowance.

Multiple Sclerosis Society of Great Britain and Northern Ireland
25 Effie Road
London SW6 1EE
Tel: 020 7736 6267

Welfare and support service for people with multiple sclerosis (MS) and their families. It has a network of 370 branches, and funds research to find the cause and cure of MS.

National Association of Councils for Voluntary Service
3rd Floor, Arundel Court
177 Arundel Street
Sheffield S1 2NU
Tel: 0114 278 6636

Promotes and supports the work of Councils for Voluntary Service.

National Association of Volunteer Bureaux
New Oxford House
16 Waterloo Street
Birmingham B2 5UG
Tel: 0121 633 4555

Information on matters related to volunteering, with a directory of volunteer bureaux and other publications.

National Asthma Campaign
Providence House
Providence Place
London N1 0NT
Tel: 020 7226 2260
Fax: 020 7704 0740

Information and support on all aspects of asthma to people with asthma, their friends, family and health professionals. It has 190 branches that organise meetings with medical speakers and raise funds for medical research.

National Care Homes Association
45–49 Leather Lane
London EC1N 7TJ
Tel: 020 7831 7090

For a list of local care homes affiliated to the Association.

National Council for Voluntary Organisations (NCVO)
Regents Wharf
8 All Saints Street
London N1 9RL
Tel: 020 7713 6161

Information on local voluntary organisations that might be able to provide help.

National Federation of Women's Institutes
104 New Kings Road
London SW6 4LY
Tel: 020 7371 9300

For details of local Women's Institutes.

Parkinson's Disease Society
215 Vauxhall Bridge Road
London SW1V 3EJ
Tel: 020 7931 8080
Helpline: 020 7233 5373 (Mon–Fri 9.30am–3.30pm)

Welfare support and advice, information and funds for research.

Princess Royal Trust for Carers
142 Minories
London EC2N 1LB
Tel: 020 7480 7788
Fax: 020 7481 4729

Aim to make it easier for carers to cope by providing information, support and practical help. The local phone book may list a branch in your area.

Samaritans
Tel: 0345 90 90 90 (a low-cost call)

Someone to talk to if you are in despair.

SCOPE (formerly the **Spastics Society**)
12 Park Crescent
London W1N 4EQ
Tel: 020 7636 5020

Works with people with cerebral palsy, their families and carers. There are over 200 local groups in England and Wales, providing care and accommodation, therapy and education, and finding employment for people with cerebral palsy.

Scottish Down's Syndrome Association
158–160 Balgreen Road
Edinburgh EH11 3AH
Tel: 0131 313 4225
Fax: 0131 313 4285

Support for people with Down's syndrome and their families. There are regional branches throughout Scotland, run by volunteers.

Scottish Spina Bifida Association
190 Queensferry Road
Edinburgh EH4 2BW
Tel: 0131 332 0743

Practical help and information to people with spina bifida and/or hydrocephalus, and their families.

Stroke Association
123–127 Whitecross Street
London EC1Y 8JJ
Tel: 020 7289 6111
Local support groups, advice and information for stroke patients and their families.

Tripscope
The Courtyard
Evelyn Road
London W4 5JL
Tel: 0345 585641 (a low-cost call)

Information about travel in London and the southwest

FURTHER READING

Better Tomorrows? by Norman Warner, published by Carers National Association, London, 1995

Caring Today: National inspection of local authority support to carers, published by the Department of Health, London, 1995

Community Care: Agenda for action. Report to the Secretary of State for Social Services by Roy Griffiths, published by HMSO, London, 1988

Directory of Grant-making Trusts 1999–2000 edited by J Davis, published by Charities Aid Foundation, West Malling, Kent, 1999

Disability Rights Handbook edited by J Patterson, published by the Disability Alliance Education and Research Association, London, 1997

A Guide to Grants for Individuals in Need edited by J Harland, published by Directory of Social Change, 1998/9

Speak Up, Speak Out: research amongst members of Carers National Association, published by Carers National Association, London, 1992

Still Battling? The Carers Act one year on, published by Carers National Association, London, 1997

What Next for Carers? Findings from the Social Services Inspectorate project 'The Way Ahead', published by the Department of Social Security, London, 1995

Leaflets and information sheets

Carers National Association:

Money Worries

Council Tax

Age Concern England:

Factsheet 18: A brief guide to money benefits

Factsheet 34: Attendance Allowance and Disability Living Allowance

(see also p 125 for information about the factsheets)

ABOUT AGE CONCERN

Working with Family Carers: A handbook for care professionals is one of a wide range of publications produced by Age Concern England, the National Council on Ageing. Age Concern cares about all older people and believes that later life should be fulfilling and enjoyable. For too many this is impossible. As the leading charitable movement in the UK concerned with ageing and older people, Age Concern finds effective ways to change that situation.

Where possible, we enable older people to solve problems themselves, providing as much or as little support as they need. Our network of 1,400 local groups, supported by 250,000 volunteers, provides community-based services such as lunch clubs, day centres and home visiting.

Nationally, we take a lead role in campaigning, parliamentary work, policy analysis, research, specialist information and advice provision, and publishing. Innovative programmes promote healthier lifestyles and provide older people with opportunities to give the experience of a lifetime back to their communities.

Age Concern is dependent on donations, covenants and legacies.

Age Concern England
1268 London Road
London SW16 4ER
Tel: 020 8765 7200
Fax: 020 8765 7211

Age Concern Scotland
113 Rose Street
Edinburgh EH2 3DT
Tel: 0131 220 3345
Fax: 0131 220 2779

Age Concern Cymru
4th Floor
1 Cathedral Road
Cardiff CF1 9SD
Tel: 029 2037 1566
Fax: 029 2039 9562

Age Concern Northern Ireland
3 Lower Crescent
Belfast BT7 1NR
Tel: 028 9024 5729
Fax 028 9023 5497

PUBLICATIONS FROM AGE CONCERN BOOKS

Money Matters

Your Rights: A guide to money benefits for older people

Sally West

Written in clear and concise language, *Your Rights* guides readers through the maze of benefits available and explains all of the main areas of interest to older people.

Please ring 020 8765 7200 for more information

Using Your Home as Capital: A guide to raising cash from the value of your home

Cecil Hinton

This best-selling book for home owners, which is updated annually, gives a detailed explanation of how to raise cash from the value of your home and obtain either a regular additional income or a lump sum.

Please ring 020 8765 7200 for more information.

Managing Other People's Money, 2nd edition

Penny Letts

It is difficult enough looking after our own money let alone managing someone else's. Fully revised and updated, the new edition examines when this need might arise and provides a step-by-step guide to the arrangements that have to be made. Adopting a clear and concise approach, topics include:

- when to take over
- the powers available
- enduring power of attorney
- the Court of Protection
- what needs to be done

Ideal for both the family carer and for legal and other advice workers, the new edition is essential reading for anyone facing this challenging situation.

£9.99   0–86242–250–7

Ethnic Elders' Benefits Handbook

Sue Ward

For many older members of ethnic minority groups, the rights to Social Security benefits will be no different from those of anyone else, if you have full UK citizenship or have spent all your working life in Britain. But for many others there are special rules to cope with an already complex system. Written in clear and concise English, this handbook is intended to help anyone from an ethnic minority understand how the system works, what their rights are and how they can claim a Social Security benefit to which they may be entitled. Topics covered include: nationality law for older people; immigration law and older people; health and social care; Social Security and people from other countries.

This book aims to help people through the maze of legal issues covering immigration and citizenship, and on related Social Security rights for those at or near pension are. It is full of advice and includes an explanation of terminology, useful publications and organisations, and relevant DSS leaflets.

£9.99   0–86242–229–9

Health and care

Health and Safety in Care Homes: A practical guide

Sarah Tullett

Health and Safety in Care Homes is a comprehensive source of practical advice and information that encourages managers and owners to assess their own health and safety provision and adapt the information provided to their own situations.

£12.99   0–86242–186–1

Know Your Medicines, 3rd edition

Pat Blair

This revised and updated edition of the popular guide explains many of the common questions older people – and those who care for them – may have about the medicines they use and how these may affect them. Written in a clear and concise way, topics include: what medicines actually do; using medicines effectively; common ailments; medicines and your body systems. This new edition will prove to be a valuable source of advice and guidance.

£7.99   0–86242–226–4

Caring for Ethnic Minority Elders: A guide

Yasmin Alibhai-Brown

A guide addressing the delivery of care to older people from ethnic minority groups, this book highlights the impact of varying cultural traditions and stresses their significance in the design of individual care packages. It looks at the broader framework of how elders receive care and then considers the requirements and experiences of ten distinct ethnic minority groups.

£14.99   0–86242–188–8

Managing CareFully: A guide for home care managers

Lesley Bell

A follow-up to the immensely successful CareFully, this handbook provides advice and guidance for managers of home care services in the private, voluntary and local authority sectors. Written in clear, jargon-free language, this book supplies detailed background information to the community care reforms and service provision.

£14.99   0–86242–185–3

If you would like to order any of these titles, please write to the address below, enclosing a cheque or money order for the appropriate amount made payable to Age Concern England. Credit card orders may be made on 020 8765 7200.

Mail Order Unit
Age Concern England
1268 London Road
London SW16 4ER

INFORMATION LINE

Age Concern produces over 40 comprehensive factsheets designed to answer many of the questions older people – or those advising them – may have, on topics such as:

- finding and paying for residential and nursing home care
- money benefits
- finding help at home
- legal affairs
- making a Will
- help with heating
- raising income from your home
- transfer of assets

Age Concern offers a factsheet subscription service that presents all the factsheets in a folder, together with regular updates throughout the year. The first year's subscription currently costs £65. Single copies (up to a maximum of five) are available free on receipt of an sae.

To order your FREE factsheet list, phone 0800 00 99 66 (a free call) or write to:

Age Concern
FREEPOST (SWB 30375)
Ashburton
Devon TQ13 7ZZ

INDEX